Foundations of Clinical Hypnosis
From Theory to Practice

Edwin K. Yager, Ph.D.

Crown House Publishing Limited
www.crownhouse.co.uk
www.chpus.com

First published by

Crown House Publishing Ltd
Crown Buildings, Bancyfelin, Carmarthen, Wales, SA33 5ND, UK
www.crownhouse.co.uk

and

Crown House Publishing Company LLC
6 Trowbridge Drive, Suite 5, Bethel, CT 06801-2858, USA
www.CHPUS.com

© Edwin K. Yager, Ph.D. 2009

The right of Edwin K. Yager to be identified as the author of this work
has been asserted by him in accordance with the Copyright, Designs
and Patents Act 1988.

All rights reserved. Except as permitted under current legislation, no part
of this work may be photocopied, stored in a retrieval system, published,
performed in public, adapted, broadcast, transmitted, recorded or reproduced
in any form or by any means, without the prior permission of the copyright
owner. Enquiries should be addressed to
Crown House Publishing Limited.

British Library Cataloguing-in-Publication Data
A catalogue entry for this book is available
from the British Library.

ISBN 978-184590122-6

LCCN 2008931998

Printed and bound in the USA

Contents

Preface

I began writing this book with two major goals in mind: (1) To provide the necessary information to clinicians who are new to the subject of hypnosis and are preparing to employ the skill in their practices, and (2) To inspire those already skilled in hypnosis to continue their training by sharing personal insights and experiences with them. In my practice as a psychologist, I have found hypnosis to be of immeasurable value in helping people to help themselves. I want to present this ancient art in the form of practical, immediately usable techniques. I want to share what I know.

I have studied, taught, and clinically employed hypnotic principles for almost 40 years, and have found their use to be an effective and efficient way to accomplish desired change. This book is the product of my ongoing study, my front-line experiences, and the conclusions I have reached in consequence of those experiences.

As clinicians, we carry an ethical obligation to provide our patients with the most effective treatments available. To do so, we must avail ourselves of current information about developments and improvements in our specialties, not with the mandate to adopt all of them, but rather to evaluate each for the benefit of our patients. This obligation applies whether our discipline is surgery, psychotherapy or general medicine, and if we are exposed to a technique that purports to improve our skills, and we are satisfied that it is appropriate, we are obliged to give it serious consideration. Hypnosis offers valuable skills to *every* clinician. A wealth of validating literature is available, published in journals of medicine, dentistry and psychology, as well as in the journals of *The American Society of Clinical Hypnosis* and *The Society for Clinical and Experimental Hypnosis*. We typically resist leaving our comfort zones, preferring to continue using the methods and techniques we were trained to use and are familiar with. Yet, after exposure, one cannot deny the advantages of hypnotic techniques. Once informed, are we not obligated to study and use them?

Part I

Background

Chapter One

Hypnosis as a Concept

My initial exposure to hypnosis was through the recorded lectures of Dave Elman (1964). I listened to them repeatedly before launching into a more expansive study, and I still comprehend hypnosis much as Elman did. His concept of hypnosis as "bypassing the critical factor" rings true as an explanation of hetero-hypnosis. However, my understanding has evolved and expanded beyond what Elman taught. In this chapter, I present my own concept, and contrast it with Elman's and those of a few other leaders in the field. Ultimately, we may reach a consensus on the subject, but we certainly have not yet done so.

Each of the authorities on the subject of hypnosis that I have read over the years has had a somewhat different understanding of the phenomenon. Moreover, each has seemingly held that understanding with strong conviction as to its accuracy. I am no different. My own comprehension of hypnotic phenomena is quite clear and I wonder that others do not understand it as I do. The viewpoints and understanding presented in this book are my own, yet they are derived from the many viewpoints of those from whom I have learned the art. They are also enhanced by my personal experience of over 30 years of study, teaching, and employing the phenomena in private practice.

A teacher of hypnotic techniques is repeatedly presented with the question "What is hypnosis?" The truth is, we can most clearly respond in the negative, stating what hypnosis is *not*. Hypnosis is *not* the state of loss of control so often portrayed by entertainers. It is *not* mysterious, threatening, disabling or unnatural. We can also safely say that it *is*, above all, a natural experience, an experience we all have many thousands of times during life without identifying it as hypnosis. The hypnotic trance may be encountered on the stage of an entertainer, in the office of a clinician, or spontaneously in a great many other situations. In fact, the trance state is only one of many hypnotic responses.

What then *is* hypnosis? I do not have a self-satisfying answer to the question. Nor do any of the many "authorities" I have studied over the years. Various theories have been proposed, yet agreement is even lacking as to a clear definition of the word "hypnosis." To say the hypnotic trance is an altered state of consciousness, which can occur with different levels of awareness, and in which the subject experiences increasing degrees of suggestibility, is to *describe* the state of hypnosis, not to *define* it. On the other hand, we do know many ways to employ hypnosis for the benefit of our patients, and perhaps that is all that really matters.

Most important, I see hypnosis as a wholly natural phenomenon. Examples of typically unrecognized phenomena associated with hypnosis include learned associations, such as the connection between fear and darkness that results in a phobia, lack of awareness of painful sensations during a traumatic event, the assimilation of values from those people we consider to be authorities (a parent, teacher, or an older child), and the experience of a distorted perception of time in various situations.

Of the many theories of hypnosis in the literature, the most satisfying theory, in my opinion, is that presented by a layman, Dave Elman (1964). Elman, now deceased, was a hypnotist-entertainer who spent the latter years of his life teaching the clinical uses of hypnosis exclusively to professionals. According to Elman, hypnosis is a mental state in which the individual is suggestible to the extent that suggestions (i.e., statements, ideas, concepts) are accepted and integrated without involving conscious, critical judgment. To this viewpoint I must add that the state is highly specific to the situation, and successful achievement of the state is dependent upon the characteristics of the individuals involved, the state of mind and mood of the subject, and the setting. Additionally, following the rationale of Elman, it seems that we are also highly suggestible – that is, that we spontaneously experience hypnosis – in several common situations. Examples include when we are in the throes of an intense emotional experience, be it fear, anger, elation or other; when we are confused; and when we are in the presence of authority, however we define that authority.

Elman's concept of hypnosis, embracing as it does the possibility of involuntary, spontaneous experiences of hypnosis, explains the etiology of many dysfunctions that were acquired in consequence of the state. Examples include phobias, obsessions, compulsions and other "learned" dysfunctions. Within Elman's concept, when acquiring the dysfunction, the individual is presumed to be in an involuntary trance state, responding to "suggestions" that are implicit in the situation and, in integrating such suggestions, incurs their influence. Elman's concept also embraces the attribute of children being the best hypnotic subjects: the younger they are the less knowledge they have available with which to exercise critical judgment. It might be said that children live in a state of hypnosis and, if this is true, it is of particular importance, as we can imagine.

The accuracy of Elman's theory is demonstrated in many situations. Hypnosis occurs when our critical judgment is bypassed, and that happens when we are experiencing an intense emotion, and it seems not to matter which emotion is being activated. Hypnosis also occurs when we are confused, and it occurs when we are in the presence of authority, whether that authority is one's mother, a teacher, a doctor or someone else. In these situations, we can internalize a concept or suggestion, making it a part of our life, doing so without using rational judgment as to its advisability, and probably without conscious awareness of doing so.

Some equate "hypnosis" with "trance." In my view, trance is actually only one of many hypnotic phenomena. Further, it also seems to me that essentially any hypnotic phenomena that can be elicited by the use of trance can also be elicited without trance. Others might say that trance is covertly elicited in the course of "apparently" working without trance, or that trance spontaneously occurs in moments of intense concentration. I cannot objectively argue with either perspective and, with respect to the clinical use of hypnosis, it doesn't matter. What matters is that hypnosis is a profoundly effective intervention that is employed in all interactions between clinician and patient, whether or not it is recognized as such.

Within the trance state we may heighten or diminish the intensity of an emotion, or of our sense of smell, or of any other of our senses. We may focus our attention *on* something, or *away from* something, simply not perceiving it. We may selectively demonstrate heightened muscular tension, or seemingly total muscular flaccidity, and this may apply to both skeletal and smooth muscle.

We may demonstrate strengths of physical or of psychic nature that are not apparent in the everyday course of living. Clearly, changes do take place as an individual slips into the trance state, changes of physical and psychological nature, changes that a sensitive clinician can utilize to the advantage of the patient, preferably with the patient's knowledge. Again, based on my understanding of the phenomena, all clinicians are presently using hypnosis, knowingly or unknowingly. I also believe that, at some level, a state of hypnosis exists in all doctor-patient interactions, if only as a consequence of the doctor being seen as an authority figure.

The clinical use of hypnotic trance, regardless of the setting, can be directed toward the treatment of symptoms (e.g., "You will never want to smoke again"), employed as an analytical tool (e.g., "Be curious and allow the memory of that event to become conscious"), or utilized simply as a psychological refuge without specific treatment objective (e.g., "Imagine a sanctuary of your choosing and be there, in that sanctuary, in total control of all you perceive"). One's clinical judgment determines which approach is most appropriate.

There is yet another highly significant phenomenon manifested in the trance state, that of permitting utilization of unconscious intelligence. The utilization of intelligence that is not immediately available to consciousness is at the heart of the teachings of Milton H. Erickson, M.D. (1989b) and others including Ernest Rossi (Erickson & Rossi, 1976). The concept of being able to "think" unconsciously is foreign to some clinicians, yet most of us can recount experiences that seem to substantiate the concept. For example, solutions to problems may be unexpectedly available upon awakening; motor functions requiring judgment, yet not requiring conscious attention, are implicit in life (e.g., many behaviors such as walking or driving an automobile are commonplace); the composition of elaborate scenarios of dreams and unexplained beliefs and values occur routinely. These are all examples of unconscious intelligence.

For those who accept the concept of unconscious intelligence, its place in therapy is seen as central. Techniques for accessing and utilizing such unconscious abilities have been taught by Erickson (1989a), Watkins (1979), Cheek (1968) and Yager (1987), among others. Hypnosis is considered as the most efficient of all techniques in facilitating these abilities.

Chapter Two

*The Language of Hypnosis**

When observing its clinical use, a person who is not well-informed about hypnosis may be confused by the language employed, impressed by the clarity of the communications, or offended by the violations of "correct" grammar that occur. The language is often not conventional, but, nevertheless, there is clear purpose behind it. Both subtle and blatant instances of such uses are included in this chapter to inform the reader and to provide a common basis of understanding for those more advanced in the field.

Although employing the principles of hypnosis does not necessarily require the use of language (any vehicle of communication can be employed), verbalization is essential in the clinical setting. As clinicians, we offer suggestions, either covertly or overtly. We guide the patient to consider possibilities and to experience life in different ways, ways that are therapeutically beneficial. We may be authoritative or we may be permissive in our approach. We sometimes take liberties with the language we use, defying customary rules of syntax and presentation. We say things that would be confusing or incomprehensible to the rationally competent individual, yet they are understood at an unconscious level by the patient in trance.

A common characteristic of hypnotic work is the necessity of bypassing conscious resistance to the experience and to the healing process that is engaged. A belief that limits the acceptance of a concept held either consciously or unconsciously, can impede or altogether derail the acceptance of suggestions that would benefit the patient. The language we use is of prime importance in bypassing such limiting beliefs when they are held consciously. For example, a patient might consciously not accept the possibility that a necessary procedure can be experienced without discomfort and, unless

---

* This chapter is influenced heavily by the teachings of Dr. Steven Bierman, and Richard Bandler and John Grinder.

that resistance is bypassed, the resistance (the non-acceptance) will prevail and the patient will be unable to alter his or her perception of the experience.

We recognize that certain individuals have influenced masses of people in profound ways through the use of language. For better or for worse, Hitler, Stalin, Churchill, King and Lincoln all used language to influence their audiences. Concepts such as implied authority, the phenomenon whereby an individual simply assumes the mantle of authority, were manifested without being verbally expressed and were therefore not resisted. In much the same way, the clinician can influence the experience of the patient, and this is especially true when the patient is in the trance state of hypnosis. Many clinicians in the field hold that the greatest value of hypnosis lies in its use without formal trance, through beneficial concepts communicated in ways that are not resisted.

In his lectures, Dr. Steve Bierman defines hypnosis as "Ideas Evoking Responses." I embrace that definition. The "Ideas" of this definition can be a product of imagination, implicit in a situation, communicated by implication, or expressly verbalized. And, whether or not the "Idea" evokes a response is determined by a complicated process of believed-in efficacy on the part of the patient, possibly further complicated by unconscious resistance to the concept. In the clinical setting, where communication is largely via words, the ideas may best be expressed in the language of hypnosis.

Patterns

Richard Bandler and John Grinder studied the work of Milton H. Erickson in an attempt to explain the mechanism whereby he had such profound influence on his patients. They presented their findings in their book *Patterns of the Hypnotic Techniques of Milton H. Erickson* (Bandler & Grindler, 1975). The following discussion is based on that work. I have taken liberties with their work, incorporating explanations of my own and extracting from the lectures of Bierman, but the fundamentals are theirs. I encourage you to read their book for further comprehension of designs for bypassing resistance. Bandler and Grinder defined the following terms:

Causal Modeling refers to relating two events by implication or by direct suggestion: *"While you sit in that chair, you can feel at ease,"* and, *"Any time you do that, you will ...."*

Specific/Non-Specific refers to the use of soft, ambiguous words in direct, specific ways: *"A* certain *degree of lightness ...."* Or *"A* particular *feeling of numbness can develop."*

Implied Contrary refers to the opposite of an imperative. *"You will ..."* is easily resisted, whereas words like "might, could, can and if" cannot be disagreed with and therefore cannot be resisted.

Transderivational Phenomena refers to a statement in which the subject must furnish an interpretation in order to attach meaning to the statement. If the subject is allowed to attach a meaning that makes sense to him or her, there will be nothing to resist: *"You don't have to feel this; you can be like a bump on a log..."* Or, *"Many people, while they are here, begin to think of places they like."*

Insert the Proper Name refers to using the subject's proper name in an indirect suggestion. *"Some people in this situation, Cathy, as they listen to me, find that time passes quickly."* Or, *"I wonder if, Pete, while you are sitting there, you can remember a time when ...."*

Selectional Restriction Violation refers to metaphors that communicate suggestions. Standard rules of language may be broken and metaphors may be used in order to evoke the desired therapeutic response. For example, *"A bicycle can have scrapes and scratches and doesn't need to feel them."* Or, *"A rock doesn't have feelings."*

Deletion refers to suggestions that allow the person to create and attach the content of the suggestion, as opposed to specifying the specific content within the suggestion. Subjects will not resist what they have supplied themselves: *"You can sit there and enjoy...."* Or, *"While you are with me you can wonder...".*

Play on Ambiguities refers to loading suggestions with words, figures of speech, or phrases that have double meanings, one that is recognized, the other having therapeutic meaning. *"Right and write, know and no, visiting relatives, the touch of a man, the feel of a sofa"* are examples. The phrase *"speaking to you as a child"* is a way to suggest age-regression. *"I want you to notice my hand me the glass"* makes no sense to rational thinking, yet makes perfect sense to the subject who is deep in a hypnotic trance; the subject can act on two meanings.

Lesser Imbedded Structures refers to the inclusion of specific, therapeutic suggestions imbedded in general suggestions, e.g., *"All muscles heal – and **the heart is a muscle**." "Your body knows exactly what it needs to do to **heal rapidly and surely**." "I'm curious if you can close your eyes and experience **the beginnings of trance**." "I'm sure you can close your eyes and **experience a reduction of this dislocation**." "I'm curious to know if you can close your eyes and **experience the absence of asthma symptoms**." "I once had a patient who said **now I can just rest**."*

Illusion of Choice refers to presupposing the outcome, an indirect way of evoking a response: *"You really were scared, **weren't you**?"* a direct implication that you are not scared now. *"Can you **pay attention**?"*

Description refers to describing what the subject is experiencing at this moment: *"As you sit there in that chair ..." "Just notice any sensation there in your eyes as you ..." "Now, here in this room, as you hear the sound of my voice ..."*

Transitional Statement refers to redirecting the attention of the subject from one thing to another in the course of leading the subject toward a therapeutic objective: *"As you sit there in that chair, aware of the pressure supporting your body, you can also become aware of a certain heaviness in your eyes."*

Prescription refers to a statement of what is to be expected: *"If you sit there in that chair with your eyes closed, you can expect to feel the pressure supporting your body."*

Good Practices

We can do good things, and we can do ill-advised things, all with good intentions. The language of hypnosis includes the words and their organization, but also specific intonation, pacing, and emphasis. A few illustrations of the constructive use of language follow:

State Ideas in Positive Language

Avoid negative words such as "don't," "won't," "never," etc. Also, strenuously avoid predicting a negative outcome. Consistently predict a positive outcome, overtly and covertly, because to do otherwise suggests a negative outcome, e.g., *"Call me tomorrow and let me know how well you feel,"* as opposed to *"Call me tomorrow if you need to."*

Pace and Lead

If it is your wish to persuade another person to your way of thinking, you can best do so by first learning about that person's position regarding the issue. Then, based on that understanding, you can join with that person and lead him or her to your way of thinking through the effective use of language. This is pacing and leading. Any other approach is apt to lead to argument. This technique of guiding patients away from dysfunctional thinking, and into functional thinking, was at the core of the work of Milton Erickson and is an effective technique of trance induction, as well as of communicating therapeutic suggestions. For example: *"While you pretend that your eyes won't open, try to open them, and notice that they will not open."*

Use of Goals in Therapy

It is always advisable to initially elicit agreement from the patient on the goals of therapy. Although you may have opinions about what "should" be done, the practice of including your opinions as goals of therapy without agreement will likely meet with resistance and consequent failure of the therapy.

Ideally, goals should be simple statements of changes required to produce the desired outcome, rather than abstract, nebulous objectives. In this way progress can be measured, and positive outcome used to further the likelihood of success in addressing the next goal.

Authoritative versus Permissive Language

Stage show hypnotists typically approach their subjects in an overtly authoritative way. Such an approach works well for a small percentage of people, but, as clinicians, we cannot afford a low percentage of success; we need an approach that will be effective for a very high percentage of our patients. Most people respond to overt authority with active resistance if not outright anger. Permissive language sidesteps most resistance, greatly improving the odds of success.

On the other hand, in certain situations, direct and even authoritative communications are indicated. We are, however, advised to limit such communications to conditions in which the patient is in a highly receptive state, for example, in a deep hypnotic trance, in a state of intense emotion, or in a state of helpless dependence. One such situation, perhaps, is a patient who is in an emergency room, frightened and injured, and being addressed by a physician.

The Use of Confusion

As mentioned previously, Dave Elman (1964) taught that people are suggestible when they are experiencing an intense emotion, when they are in the presence of authority, or when they are confused. Such confusion may arise spontaneously, as in the case of a not-understood, compulsive behavior, or may be engineered for therapeutic purposes by the clinician. Self-contradictory statements expressed with sincerity, so-called "word salads" that only sound as if they have meaning, and strong words expressed in gentle ways, are among the verbal ways of creating confusion. Their use can set the stage for the covert introduction of suggestions for a trance experience, or for altered perception of an undesired stimulus such as an injection or suturing procedure.

The Use of Verbal Cues

The most effective hypnotic suggestions include cues, cues that prescribe when the suggestions are to be effective. Cues can be verbal or nonverbal; they can be any event, a time of day, a thought, or an experience. The suggestion, *"You will feel hungry"* is not a complete suggestion; it needs a cue. Cues are automatically inserted when you begin a suggestion with the word "When." Whatever follows that word becomes the cue of the suggestion. An example of a verbal cue is, *"Be curious to see what happens when I say the word 'now'."* An example of a nonverbal cue would be, *"Be curious to see what happens when the bell rings."*

The Use of Voice Shifts

Variations in intensity, emotional expression, and emphasis through changes in volume or tone, can all be utilized to covertly underscore a clinically significant portion of a suggestion. The true meaning of a suggestion can thus be communicated without conscious attention, as that could inspire resistance.

Designing Direct Hypnotic Suggestions

Hypnotic suggestions are:

Brief, concise expressions
that
use the language of hypnosis
to
communicate desired outcome
and are
phrased in consonant words
that
bypass resistance
and
may not conform to conventional rules of syntax, grammar
and punctuation.

Usually, hypnotic suggestions should:

Be phrased permissively
using
soft, gentle words
that
communicate concepts understandable to the patient,
expressed in language understandable to the patient.

Occasionally, hypnotic suggestions may:

Be phrased forcefully
using
strong, commanding words
that
communicate concepts understandable to the patient,
expressed in language understandable to the patient.

Examples of using permissive gentle words versus forceful, commanding words:

"May," versus "Will"
"You may find it true," versus "You are finding it true."
"Perhaps there will be a tingling feeling," versus "You will feel a tingling feeling."
"You may find your eyes are glued closed," versus "Your eyes are glued closed."
"Permit yourself to sleep now," versus "Sleep!"
"Allow your hand to rise," versus "Raise your hand."
"Become aware of the change," versus "Pay attention to the change."

Examples of using consonant words versus harsh, abrasive words:

"Close your eyes," versus "Shut your eyes."
"Your eyes are glued closed," versus "You can't open your eyes."
"You may notice discomfort," versus "You may feel pain."
"You may feel pressure," versus "You may feel a moment of sharp pain."
"You may be experiencing difficulty," versus "You are having a problem."
"Nothing to bother, nothing to disturb," versus "I'll be giving you a shot now."
"Call to let me know how well you are doing," versus "Call me when something goes wrong."
"You will awaken feeling hungry," versus "You will awaken without the need to vomit."

***

The language of hypnosis, when fully embraced by a clinician, can be an influential means of covertly communicating suggestions, engendering compliance, and otherwise enhancing the doctor-patient relationship. It is facilitated effectively by first comprehending the concepts involved, followed by the premeditated practice of those concepts.

Chapter Three

The Phenomena of Hypnosis

Miracles happen, not in opposition to Nature,
but in opposition to what we know of Nature.

St. Augustine

Talking about hypnosis is like talking about the ether: there are no objective "handles" to use. There is not even an agreed-upon definition, and no adjectives are available that adequately describe the state of mind that evolves. We can only relate some of the phenomena, physical and mental, that are associated with the state, to the state some authorities refer to as "trance." In this chapter, I describe the essential phenomena of hypnosis.

Hypnosis is not only a natural experience, it is an intrinsic part of our lives. On many occasions we spontaneously go into the state of mind that is best defined as trance. Examples include the remarkable recovery of the child who has banged a knee and comes crying to Mother, and upon Mother's kiss is magically soothed; the mystical power of the placebo effect; and, as an example on the negative side, the mystery of how an intelligent, thinking person can convince himself or herself that the bitter taste of tobacco smoke is enjoyable. Any time our attention is strongly focused, or any time our emotions are powerfully aroused, we are in a state of mind that can be identified as hypnosis.

Trance is but one hypnotic phenomenon. Because trance is so natural an experience, one of the most common post-trance responses in the clinical setting from subjects who have experienced it for the first time, is to question whether they actually experienced hypnosis at all. It was not what they expected – therefore they wonder if anything indeed happened. They often use expressions such as, "I don't believe I was hypnotized" and "I heard every word you said."

Since it often seems important for patients to have a sense of having experienced the state, I elaborate on the naturalness of hypnosis in advance of guiding them into trance. Then, to ratify the experience as much as possible, I guide them by suggesting that they experience some trance phenomena such as levitating a hand, accessing a very early memory, or eliciting an ideomotor response to a question.

In response to suggestions, a person may be subjectively aware of the elicited hallucinations, abreactions, or physical stimulation. Also, one may be aware of the hypersensitivity of the senses, such as hearing a whispered conversation on the other side of the room, or becoming aware of one's own heartbeat. On the other hand, in response to suggestions, the subject may be *unaware* of, or unresponsive to, stimulation of any of the senses.

The Issue of Control

Fear of hypnosis is the most common barrier to be overcome in the clinical situation. If the patient is preoccupied with thoughts about negative possibilities, such thoughts *will* interfere with achieving the trance state. The clinician is advised to identify any concerns the patient has before trance is attempted, and to provide adequate explanation and reassurance, so that the patient can achieve and enjoy the benefits of the trance state.

Patients who are considering hypnosis for the first time are often worried about loss of control. When asked about their impressions of hypnosis, these people will point to concerns about being under the control of someone else, or being asleep or unconscious, or other mistaken ideas that may seem threatening. Entertainers and others in the entertainment media who employ hypnosis contribute to this misperception by presenting the interaction as a master–slave relationship. The net result is an unfortunate and inaccurate understanding of a wholly natural experience, an experience that occurs spontaneously, and one that can have remarkable clinical value.

The information most commonly missing is that *the subject is aware of what is happening*. Were the subject not aware, communication would not be possible. Yes, inhibitions are reduced in trance, and yes, the subject is more suggestible, but he or she is not actually under the arbitrary control of another person unless further deception is employed.

Yet even today a debate on the question of control is in full swing. There are those who maintain that a subject will not do anything that is against personal morals or convictions, and that the subject is in fact in control when the chips are down. Skeptics point to examples that appear to be evidence to the contrary: the Jim Jones mass suicide, Hitler's and Stalin's exploits, and the success of the CIA in creating the ideal assailant that have recently come to light. Attempts to clarify the question by controlled experiment have not proved convincing. How can one design such an experiment? The problems encountered in designing good research in this area seem to lie in the near impossibility of controlling, or even identifying, all of the variables involved. We must rely on historical, and often anecdotal, experience, and that is not satisfying to the skeptics.

I usually address the question in my classes on hypnosis by conducting a demonstration that affords the opportunity to raise the question in a dramatic manner, but without resolution.

> I guide a volunteer to experience trance, then guide him or her to experience arm levitation. Further, I suggest that the subject's arm will rise promptly every time I tug on my earlobe, and return to resting when I scratch my leg, and that this will be true even after rousing from trance, and even though the suggestion is not consciously remembered. (This last addition is, of course, a covert, and relatively ineffective, suggestion for amnesia for the suggestion itself.) Assuming the basic suggestion is accepted and followed, and it usually is, I exercise the cues to the great amusement of the class. Then I ask the subject, *"Who is in control of your arm?"* The initial response is usually "I am," whereupon I will repeat the sequence of ear tug and leg scratch and inquire again. At some point, the demonstration subject also begins to express reservations regarding the question, at which point I say, in an authoritative, almost commanding way, *"I want you to take control of that arm now – within your own mind – in your own way."* Upon again exercising the cue, there is no response.

> I then point out that control was regained at my suggestion and perhaps, if that is true – if I have the power to *give* control – perhaps

at some meta-level I have the power to take it away again. Then, having implied that I have resumed the power, I tug at my earlobe and the levitation usually recurs.

By this point, confusion is apparent in the class and I leave the students with the confusion. Experience has taught me that, by the next class session the authority of the suggestion will have expired, so I am not concerned about lasting effect. I just want the students to ponder the issue of control and to consider the ethical implications associated with the issue.

It is the issue of control and the associated moral and ethical implications that are of concern to me. I do not want control. I do not want the responsibilities that would accompany control, and I do not believe it would be in the best interest of the patient for him or her ever to relinquish control, even if it were possible. By pre-hypnotic suggestion, direct suggestions during trance, and by post-hypnotic suggestions, I state, imply, and emphasize the concept that the patient is in control. By doing so, I believe the concept is adequately reinforced. And yet I cannot help but wonder about the potential power of the link between "influence" and "control."

Expectation

For me, the word "expectation" provides a satisfying explanation for our experiences. It seems that we usually experience what we *expect* to experience, be it pain, joy or grief. A mother-to-be can have an easy, normal delivery if that is what she expects to have, and a traumatic delivery if she expects it to be traumatic; an athlete who expects to perform well will do so, and will perform poorly if that is expected. In addition, expectation seems to have a place in experience that is different from belief. I may believe that I have the ability to demonstrate some unusual physical feat, but somehow that is only theoretical and, unless I *expect* to be able to do it, I will likely not succeed. Thanks to their expectations, subjects in trance are able to do many things they would not be able to do in the normal waking state. For example, suspended between two chairs by the shoulders and feet, a slight female can support the weight of a heavy male sitting on her midsection. Such subjects may also be able to remember long-forgotten events with remarkable clarity, and to dissociate, hallucinate and perform mysterious feats of mental gymnastics as well. It would seem that it is the task of the clinician to guide the subject to *expect* the suggested event will occur and, if the *clinician* expects to be successful in doing so, the communication of expectation will usually come to pass. A major aspect of training in the use of hypnosis lies in providing a clinician with experiences that lead to such expectation.

Conditioning

It is apparent that people are conditioned by life experiences, and it is often by means of hypnotic phenomena that conditioning happens. Small children live in a state definable as trance, and a child who is demeaned by defeating statements from someone in a position of perceived authority such as "You are so dumb!" and "You'll never amount to anything!", will almost certainly be conditioned to limit his or her performance. Moreover, unless reconditioning occurs, this conditioning will have lifelong influence. It is no accident that Christian parents usually have Christian children, and that Moslem parents have Moslem children. We believe what we were conditioned to believe; we have skills and limitations we were conditioned to have. More about conditioning is to come in following chapters.

Suggestibility

There is little doubt that we are more suggestible while in trance than in the normal waking state. Entertainers demonstrate this dramatically, and clinicians familiar with its use endorse the fact. Yet, what do we mean by the word "suggestible?"

Dave Elman (1964) spoke of being suggestible as a state of mind in which we are able to integrate a suggestion – embracing it and making it a part of our life's experience – and doing so without exercising critical judgment about its appropriateness or advisability. This notion of suggestibility provides an explanation for our susceptibility to influences that covertly affect us. Moreover, it seems that we spontaneously experience states of suggestibility many hundreds of times in life. We are suggestible when in an intense emotional state, and it doesn't seem to matter which emotion we are experiencing. We are suggestible when we are confused. We are suggestible in the presence of authority, whatever we consider authority to be. In other words, hypnosis is a universally experienced, natural phenomenon that is an ongoing element of life.

A child who has not yet learned enough about life to be capable of critically judging the content of a suggestion, whether communicated by means of words or implicit in the situation, might be said to live in a state of hypnosis. Perhaps that is why it seems so very important to restrict what the child is exposed to. To most young children there is no higher authority than "Mom," a concept that is usually modified with maturity. A second-grader may integrate the concept that math is difficult if that concept is presented by an authoritative third-grader – and that influence may prevail thereafter, limiting the child's ability to perform well in that area.

The door of suggestibility permits the entrance of desired change if properly approached. It also permits the entrance of undesired change; it permits the "learning" of behaviors, beliefs and experience that become dysfunctional in later life, such as phobias, destructive habits and self-demeaning convictions. Compulsions, obsessions, dissociative issues, hypertension, irritable bowel, tension and migraine headaches, many dermatological problems, and asthma also fall into this list of examples. However, suggestibility also permits the entrance of desired change.

Hypnotic Susceptibility

Many attempts have been made to measure hypnotic susceptibility. Most are based on the theory that there is an enduring human trait – a susceptibility to experience hypnosis. Scales have been designed in attempts to quantify this parameter, examples of which include the *Stanford Hypnotic Susceptibility Scale, Harvard Group Scale, Stanford Group Scale, Psychological Absorption Scale* and *the Differential Attentional Process Inventory Scale*. These scales all share a common theme: The subject is first exposed to a trance induction procedure, then a series of suggestions are given and the responses to these suggestions are recorded. In theory, the higher the response score, the greater the susceptibility of the subject.

We are all highly susceptible in some situations, and the younger we are, the more susceptible we are likely to be. We may be very responsive when guided by one individual and not by another. We may be responsive at one time, or in one situation, or in one mood, and not in others. Although the susceptibility scales may have value for research purposes, I consider them to be of no value clinically, and even of negative value if the clinician limits the use of hypnosis based on performance on the scales: the patient might perform well in addressing clinical material, even though not performing on the scale. Our degree of susceptibility depends upon multiple factors and with practice and conditioning we can improve our skill at experiencing hypnosis.

Our degree of susceptibility depends upon multiple factors. Bowers (1976) suggests that we can improve our skill at experiencing hypnosis by training in hypnosis, or simply by practice and by using biofeedback.

My favorite illustration of a non-quantified test of hypnotic susceptibility is that taught by Milton Erickson. Facing the subject, he would ask in his slowly paced voice, "What do you see over here?" while simultaneously slowly gesturing by moving his relaxed, open hand from his body sideways to full-arm extension. According to Dr. Erickson, the subject who responds, "your hand" is a good subject, whereas the subject who responds, "the table, window, door" or whatever is over here, is not. As I understand the dynamics of the test, it is the sensitivity of the subject to the word "here" versus the nonverbal communication reflected in the gesture that is the discernment. While I do not doubt that the test had value for Dr. Erickson, I have not found it personally to be of value.

The Nocebo Response

The nocebo is the clinical reciprocal of the placebo and is illustrated by the following examples.

- Volunteers were told a mild electrical shock would be passed through their heads and might cause a headache. No electrical current was actually passed, but two-thirds of them developed a headache (Hahn, 1997).

- Patients with asthma were divided into two groups. One was given a bronchoconstrictor, which ordinarily makes symptoms worse, and was told it was a bronchodilator, which normally improves the symptoms. This placebo suggestion reduced their discomfort by nearly 50%. The second group was given a bronchodilator and told it was a bronchoconstrictor. The nocebo suggestion reduced the drug's effectiveness by nearly 50% (Spiegel, 1997).

- The same treatment can work as both a nocebo and placebo. Experimenters gave subjects who believed they were allergic to various foods an injection which they were told contained the allergen. It was only salt water, but it produced allergic symptoms in many of the subjects. The experimenters injected salt water again, this time saying it would neutralize the effect of the previous injection – and in many cases it did (Spiegel, 1997).

- An active drug has more nocebo power than a mere sugar pill. In one study, experimental subjects were divided into four groups. The first group was given a muscle relaxant, described correctly; the second group was given the same muscle relaxant but was told it was a stimulant; the third group received a sugar pill described as a muscle relaxant, and the fourth received the same inert pill described as a stimulant (Barsky et al., 2002; Bellamy, 1997; Beneditti et al., 2003).

  To no one's surprise, subjects who thought the pill was a stimulant were more likely to say they felt tense. But the muscle relaxant caused more reports of tension when described as a stimulant than the sugar pill did. Blood levels of the muscle relaxant were lower in people told it was a stimulant than those told the truth. They may have absorbed less of the drug because the false information activated the sympathetic nervous system, which slows down movements of the intestinal tract.

Trance Phenomena

Abreaction

Although there is not universal agreement on the definitions of several hypnotic terms, including "abreaction", the term is used here to identify that condition in which a subject is *re-experiencing* a past event, as opposed to *remembering* the event. Not only does visual recall occur in abreaction, but also the experience of emotion and all of the senses, just as if the event were happening in the present.

Clinically, the term "abreaction" is used to describe the experience of *re-living* an event in the course of remembering it. In this situation, all of the senses that were activated in the original experience are activated in the present, and the patient will demonstrate this physically. Moreover, the patient will experience the event in real time – the phenomenon of time-distortion is not apparent. A classic illustration of these phenomena is the experience of patients undergoing Primal Therapy, as taught by Janov.

In the 1950s, Janov made quite a splash in the waters of psychotherapy by introducing and promoting what he called "Primal Therapy." By the use of hypnotic techniques, he was able to demonstrate abreaction to the birth experience, and the sights and sounds of the resultant performance were impressive to the most skeptical observer. The sight of a grown man curled into the fetal position and squalling like a newborn infant gave rise to considerable publicity. This "therapy" lost popularity and lost credibility as a valid intervention because – despite its dramatic appeal to many – it simply did not produce desired change. The technique was, nevertheless, a clear demonstration of abreaction; the exercise was not therapeutic, only abreactive.

In my view, abreaction is contraindicated in all but a few clinical situations because of the risks of reinforcing the negative influence of the initial event and the breakdown of a distressed patient. It is additionally contraindicated because of the fact that any work must be done in real time, thereby prolonging therapy. Abreaction could, however, be indicated in a situation where an emotionally stable patient would benefit from the greater wealth of information available while abreacting. Offsetting the risk of reinforcing negative influence, it is also true that the patient may obtain additional understanding of an event which has not been available by other means and thus get information that is vital to the resolution of a problem. Again, we find clinical judgment must prevail.

Eliciting abreaction of an event may be accomplished by direct suggestion for the experience, as in, *"As I touch your hand, you are there, in that dark closet."* Alternatively, abreaction may be elicited by phrasing the suggestion for a memory using verbs in the present tense. For example, *"You* are *there,"* as opposed to, *"You* were *there."* Additionally, abreaction can occur spontaneously, as sometimes happens during emotionally laden interviews.

Absence of Voluntary Activity

The absence of voluntary activity is another physical change associated with trance. In the usual clinical situation, as the patient slips into the trance state, an absence of physical movement becomes apparent. On stage with an entertainer, the subjects may (with the nonverbal encouragement of the entertainer) lean on each other. In the office of a clinician, a male patient, for example, relaxes his skeletal muscles and remains apparently immobile. The patient knows he can move; he just doesn't want to. The patient has not been deprived of the ability to control skeletal muscle; he is just not inclined to do anything.

In the normal waking state we are in almost constant motion. We may smile, frown, scratch, gesture or shift position. We may look around, swallow or move in some other way. Yet, when in trance, we display almost no motion at all, and the clinician can ratify the trance state for the patient by pointing out the lack of motion to the patient.

In some medical situations it is necessary to immobilize a patient. In such cases, the use of trance can be adequate for extended periods of time or, alternatively, can provide immobility of selected bodily areas by suggestion.

Access to Unconscious Intelligence

Although contested by some clinicians, an unconscious domain of the mind appears to exist that is separate and distinct from consciousness. Arguments for this concept are based on the following, definable parameters:

1. The task of regulating the bodily functions that maintain life, (respiration, digestion, blood chemistry, glandular function, etc.), is beyond conscious capacity to comprehend, much less to control the required musculature every minute of every day. Moreover, we have essentially no conscious awareness of any aspect of that process.

2. Memory itself seems to be a process of communication from the unconscious domain to consciousness, through the vehicle of our senses. Although we are not accustomed to being aware of this process, we have the ability to become aware of it. For example, we can perceive how the spelling of the word "cat" is communicated from the unconscious to conscious domains when we are asked for the spelling. The reader is encouraged to pause for a moment to subjectively experience the phenomenon. Some people "see" the letters in their mind's eye; others may "hear" the letters being spoken. When we recall the appearance of some person in our past, we consciously "see" an image of the person in our mind's eye. When we recall the sound of something in our past, we consciously "hear" that sound.

Yet there is far more persuasive evidence of unconscious capacities. In the course of developing the concept of Subliminal Therapy (see Chapter 12), assumptions of unconscious abilities and organization have proved to be valid. Those assumptions have been tested clinically and support without question that such unconscious intelligence exists, separate and apart from consciousness. Moreover, it can be enlisted for therapeutic purpose. The trance state most effectively provides access to that intelligence, and patients will consistently spontaneously enter trance in the course of employing Subliminal Therapy.

Age Regression

As used here, this term refers to *remembering* a past event, without *reexperiencing* the event. In illustration, although a female subject, for example, may remember what she had for breakfast, she is aware that she is not having breakfast right now (see "abreaction" for the contrasting experience).

Anesthesia and Analgesia

"Anesthesia" is defined as a complete lack of awareness of experience; "analgesia" is defined as awareness of what is happening without sensitivity to physical stimulus. Either condition is available by suggestion to a responsive subject who is in trance.

The Use of Dissociation

Each of us has likely experienced a feeling of unreality at some time, in some situation. When analyzed, such an experience will conform to theories of dissociation. As is demonstrable in hypnotic trance, having an arm that is intellectually recognized as being present (because you can *see* it and *move* it), but which is subjectively devoid of awareness in a tactile sense, is a confusing and educational experience. It is through this phenomenon that the woman in the delivery room is able to participate and cooperate in the birth, aware of all that is happening, but protected from physical sensation of a negative sort. An additional illustration is that acts of heroism in war are normally accompanied by an indifference to pain or other stimulation, just as accident victims are often unaware of the extent of their injury.

There are various reports of dissociative experiences in the literature: near-death reports often include out-of-body perception, and hypnotic recall of surgical procedures involving general anesthesia are most often reported from a perspective of being above the table. Then too, dreams are often replete with self-observance from a perspective outside of the self. Premeditated, specific dissociation of experience by suggestion lies within the domain of trance work.

Attachment of emotion: Although dissociation from emotion is a common experience while in trance, usually occuring without suggestions being offered, it is also possible for a subject to selectively experience an emotion when it is suggested. This step might be indicated where a patient would benefit from the additional understanding afforded.

Dissociation from emotion: A patient presenting an intense state of anxiety will normally be relieved of that anxiety while in trance. In like form, states of depression, grief, anger and other emotions can be set aside for the period of the trance.

We speak of hypnosis in terms of dissociation, with the ability of a subject "to get away from" emotional influences as a hallmark of the state, and this is an exceedingly valuable aspect for clinical purposes. A depressed, anxious or otherwise disabled patient is unable to think clearly, and analytic ability is compromised with consequent jeopardy to any decisions made. By guiding the patient to experience trance, the clinician enables a state in which the patient can more objectively evaluate problems and reach realistic conclusions. By teaching the patient the skill of self-hypnosis, the clinician enhances the patient's ability to mitigate the symptoms (the physical reactions to the emotions). The duration of such relief will vary substantially from patient to patient, but can always be reinforced by further trance experience.

Dissociation from cognitive function: The experience of trance is not consistent from person to person. While one may report it as being very similar to the normal waking state, another will report it as being dream-like, and still another as being somewhere in space. Clearly, suggestion will influence the experience; however, even without suggestion there is substantial variance. There is usually a disinclination to engage in analytical or reasoning activity, and a clear disinterest in social involvement. Another indication of dissociation of cognition is that following the experience of trance some patients will be unable to recall events that occurred during the period of the trance. When questioned, some will spontaneously report having no memory of having had the experience at all, or perhaps vehemently claim that the event never happened.

Focus and Defocus of Attention

Focusing attention is an essential element of all trance inductions. It is also a characteristic of the state achieved in that the patient's focus is directed by suggestion. For example, a patient can be guided to focus attention *on* something to the exclusion of other awareness. In this manner, an uncomfortable stimulus can become a matter of indifference while attention is focused on a pleasant stimulus.

The patient can also be guided to focus attention *away from* an uncomfortable stimulus and, in the right situation, a skilled clinician can provide relief more effectively than is available from medications. This "right situation" depends on many elements, certainly including the influence of well-intended comments and suggestions from other attending personnel, ability to consider non-traditional concepts, and freedom from distracting events.

Hallucination

In trance, any of the senses can be hallucinated, alone or in combination with other senses, and they may be hallucinated either positively or negatively. This ability can be of marked value in psychotherapy. Suggestions can be vividly implanted by guiding the patient to imagine a desired situation, engaging all possible senses to make the imagined situation "real." By embracing visual imagery in combination with auditory, kinesthetic and olfactory elements, the imagined situation can subjectively become exceedingly real, and therefore have greater influence.

Hyper- and Hyposensitivity to Stimuli

A subject in trance can be guided to *hear* a whispered conversation that others are not even aware exists, or may be guided to *not hear* the sound of a loud noise in the immediate vicinity. It is all a matter of suggestion, and any or all of the senses can be so influenced.

Increased/Decreased Muscle Strength

By means of suggestion to a subject in trance, his or her physical strength may be either enhanced or compromised. Stage entertainers demonstrate this phenomenon as they alternately enhance the strength of an outstretched arm, and then take away that strength. It is similarly demonstrated when the entertainer suggests that the subject will be unable to stand (or otherwise move), and by the semi-paralysis sometimes spontaneously experienced in a state of panic.

Relaxation of Musculature

As we enter trance, some changes consistently and spontaneously take place: some are physical and some are mental. One of the more obvious physical changes is that the musculature of the body is relieved of tension. This release of muscular tension is apparent to the subject when the therapist suggests *"Any place in your body where you focus your attention, you can be aware of the release of tension that has taken place there."* Such guided attention affirms the trance experience and is reassuring to the patient.

Although not subjectively apparent to the patient, the clinician should be aware that the release of tension applies not only to skeletal muscle, but to smooth muscle as well. It may be advantageous to point this out to the patient in the form of a mini-lecture about the function of smooth muscle in the digestive process, the respiratory process, the control of the pattern of blood flow in the body, and that the glands themselves are ducts lined with smooth muscles. The clinician should also point out that although we have voluntary control of skeletal muscle we do not have voluntary control of smooth muscle. For example, we cannot consciously stop the process of digestion. It is, however, true that we can at least *influence* smooth musculature and that an effective way to do so is through the use of hypnosis. The clinician should also point out to the patient that our bodies respond physically to what we experience emotionally, that lists of physical changes have been compiled corresponding to various emotional states, and that such changes, experienced on a protracted basis, would be diagnosed as a physical illness. This also becomes a rational explanation for the psychogenesis of many illnesses.

Release of Inhibition

The outlandish antics of volunteers in stage demonstrations of hypnosis seem amazing; it seems unreasonable that reasonable people would behave in such ways. This is an illustration of the release of inhibition that characterizes trance – the subjects are freer to dance and sing and have fun. This release of inhibition is of obvious value to the entertainer, and it is also of value to the clinician because patients are freer to recall and discuss unpleasant memories, and even to engage in treatment at all. One explanation for the phenomenon of reduced inhibition is that it relates to the dissociation from emotion as discussed above; embarrassment, like other emotions, is simply not experienced.

Time Compression and Time Expansion

Time distortion is an inherent characteristic of the trance state. Patients are often surprised at how rapidly a hypnotic session went by. This capacity for time distortion can be used advantageously in the clinical setting and is accomplished by suggestion. A suggestion for review of a large number of memories, covering an extensive time span, will probably produce that result. Also, suggestion for leisurely or detailed review will likely be successful.

In fact, the patient can be guided to *"slowly review the memory of some experience, examining each detail as it passes."* This latter option is of particular value in the forensic use of hypnosis, in which a witness is interviewed while in trance when all possible details are desired.

In the medical domain, a patient can utilize time compression to subjectively compress, in time, an uncomfortable period of healing, or an uncomfortable procedure. Simultaneously, the patient can remain sensitive to, and retain the benefits of, any positive elements experienced, such as affirmative comments made by the physician or the attending staff.

Subjectively Experienced Trance Phenomena

As mentioned in the beginning of this chapter, one of the more common reactions of those who experience trance for the first time is to honestly question whether they experienced trance at all; the experience is subjectively natural, and objective measures of difference are lacking. Yet, trance does offer potentially dramatic differences in subjective experience, ranging from abreaction of past events to hallucinated events and experience.

Milton Erickson (1960) spoke of the marked differences in the sense of reality of the person in trance. He alluded to a shift from awareness of external reality to an awareness of internal reality. The subject in trance becomes relatively indifferent to external stimuli and so is less responsive to them. From the perspective of the subject, this change in reality may not be consciously recognized at the time; however, it may be recognized during post-trance review of the experience.

Observable Trance Phenomena

Several physical changes are objectively observable and are typically demonstrated by a subject in trance. These signs, enumerated below, can be of value to the therapist by indicating when succeeding steps should be accomplished, or, for the practitioner just beginning to use hypnosis, by providing essential feedback supporting induction success, i.e., a test. While these signs are involuntary, not all will always be present; it is a pattern of such signs that is indicative of trance.

Eye Changes

Our eyes are the most sensitive organs of our bodies and therefore it is not surprising that change would occur there. Most subjects will roll their eyes upward under the eyelids during the induction of trance and maintain them in that position during trance. This upward roll can be observed by the deformation of the eyelids as the eye rolls upward. It is, of course, true that this upward roll is usually observed in natural sleep; however, it is easily demonstrated as an uncomfortable position to maintain in the waking state.

If open, the eyes typically become fixed in orientation, with a defocused appearance, and the frequency of eye blink will be sharply reduced. Also, eye flutter is common, especially as the subject begins to close them, and may continue for some time thereafter.

Absence of Volitional Activity

It is highly likely that the adult in trance will sit or lie motionless. On the other hand, the child will scratch, gesture, wiggle and laugh aloud in an almost normal manner. I have no firm explanation for this difference; however, it may simply be that the adult knows what is expected, whereas a child may not. For adults, this characteristic can be of value in the medical setting where it is desirable that the patient remains motionless for extended periods of time.

Muscular Relaxation

This change is obvious to the observer and to the subject alike. All skeletal muscles of the body are permitted to release tension and to become flaccid, and the depth of trance is correlated with the degree of relaxation. Moreover, the release of tension applies to smooth musculature as well. It is my unsubstantiated opinion that the dissociation of emotion associated with trance is responsible for this release of tension. Essential smooth muscle function is not impeded, and abnormal blood pressure, respiration and glandular function will usually and promptly return to baseline as the patient enters trance. However, regardless of the basis of the change, the release is apparent to the patient and observer alike. Moreover, prompting the subject to be aware of the release is a way to ratify the experience of trance for the subject.

Pattern of Breathing Shifts to Diaphragmatic

This is an easily observed change. The rise and fall of the chest with breathing substantially diminishes and abdominal rise and fall becomes apparent.

Conservation of Energy

Usually, voice volume will be lowered and speech slowed, sometimes requiring the therapist to move closer to the subject to hear the words being spoken. Responses to questions will be brief and not elaborated upon unless there is a specific request or suggestion. If the question, "Do you know what time it is?" is asked of a person in the normal waking state, the answer will probably be a statement of the time. Asked of the person in trance, the answer will probably be "yes" or "no." This characteristic relates to the absence of voluntary movement, although it may manifest in slowed thinking as well, if not countermanded by suggestion.

Absence of the Swallow Reflex

Salivation is usually depressed in trance; therefore swallowing will correspondingly be absent.

Waking Hypnosis

Many authorities in the field have stated that any hypnotic phenomenon, or any behavior, that can be elicited in trance can be elicited without trance.

It depends, I suppose, on how hypnosis and trance are defined. Is the individual in the emergency room for repair of a serious injury in trance? Is a child who is terrified at having been threatened by an animal in trance? Is the accident victim, lying on the freeway with a compound fracture, in trance? Clearly, it can be argued that they are all in trance. What about the guy being questioned by a traffic officer? Or the patient listening to the doctor describe how to exercise a sore joint? Or the prospective customer listening to a used car salesman? Or the child listening to his irate mother?

In my classes, usually on the first day, I typically demonstrate waking hypnosis by selecting an accessible male with hairy arms and asking his permission to use him as a demonstration subject. Having obtained permission, I say to him, "*In a moment, I am going to stroke this arm three times, lightly and distinctly, and you will then find that nothing I do will bother or disturb you.*" I then slowly stroke his arm, maintaining eye contact and speaking with authority, "Nothing to bother, and nothing to disturb." Having completed the stroking, I will then use my thumb and forefinger to pull some hair from his arm and sprinkle the hair so the class can see it. The look of surprise on the face of the subject, combined with his (usual) verbal expressions of disbelief, constitutes convincing evidence to the class that formally induced trance is not necessary to experience hypnosis.

Yet, on reconsideration, trance was likely present. I am a large man and as I approached the seated male, he must have felt somewhat defenseless in the situation. Permission was given to refuse to be a subject, yet it would have been awkward for him to have refused permission, and he must have been wondering about what I intended to do. All of the ingredients for trance induction were present: his attention was focused, my bearing was authoritative, and I voiced a suggestion in a context in which he could not resist. True, he never closed his eyes, he didn't relax significantly, and he may have demonstrated a sense of humor, but none of those are prerequisites for trance.

Perhaps it would be more accurate to say that anything that can be accomplished following a formal trance induction can be accomplished without such formality.

Ideo-responses

As I wrote the words you are reading, my fingers selected and pressed the keys on my computer keyboard, all without conscious attention or control. Similarly, when I stood and walked away, my limbs functioned without conscious decisions about which leg to move in what direction. I *learned* these functions, initially through conscious volition. The behaviors were then relegated to unconscious control.

The term "ideomotor response" has been used to define such functioning; however, in the discipline of hypnotic work, the term has a different meaning. As opposed to cognitively learned behavior, it refers to the communication of meaningful intelligence from the unconscious domain of the mind by means of coded physical movements. Examples include the use of finger signals, as most significantly taught by Dr. David Cheek (1994), the use of a pendulum in which the direction of swing is coded to have specific meaning, automatic writing, and the Ouija Board – that old game still-popular in toy stores.

We play with Ouija Boards and are mystified – and sometimes frightened – by them. Mystics sometimes use pendulums to impress their clients, and finger signals are used by highly respected clinicians. Such phenomena are fascinating to some, frightening to some, seen as evidence of evil by others, and yet all can be employed for constructive purpose. We can pose questions to our unconscious mind and receive answers that may be of value. We also can often determine the acceptability of a suggestion that has been posed.

These phenomena are evidence of unconscious intelligence. The intelligence required to regulate bodily functioning in ways that sustain life is beyond our conscious capacity to comprehend. The first small step is to realize that unconscious intelligence has the ability to communicate meaningfully. The only problem with utilizing such communications in therapy lies in the time-consuming process of preparing the communication. It is far more efficient to utilize an inner voice or visualization technique. And yet, at the same time, it is subjectively impressive to a patient to experience the involuntary swing of a pendulum, or the lifting of a finger that has meaning associated with the motion. It somehow carries conviction and may be used to confirm, deny or question conscious opinion.

Chapter Four

The Tools of Hypnosis

Remembering is an awakening,
Progressively feeling alive,
As I shed the protective oblivion,
I once needed to survive.

Barbara Tierney, 2007

There are many different hypnotic phenomena, and many ways to utilize each of them. An extensive range of tools is available to the clinician. Each tool has its own possibilities and limitations, and each will be valuable in particular situations. The clinician's challenge is to select the most appropriate phenomenon for the situation at hand, ensuring that the chosen phenomenon will be for the benefit of the patient.

Trance

Although some may be surprised, I would include trance as a tool of hypnosis. I do so because the trance state is but one of many hypnotic phenomena. Most, if not all, demonstrations of hypnotic effects can be accomplished without a formal trance induction, although the trance state may facilitate any or all such effects. Clinically, a primary purpose of trance is to enhance authority, thereby enhancing responsiveness to suggestions and providing access to capabilities that are not available in the normal waking state.

A person in the trance state exhibits distinct changes, as discussed in Chapter 3, and some of these changes afford opportunities that are of clinical value. Dissociation from emotional influence and enhanced memory capacity are among the most valuable of these changes.

Suggestion

It is important to recognize the significance of the word "suggestion." It does not embrace authority, such as "command" would convey. Instead, it offers the option of rejecting its content. Yet, the history of hypnosis is fraught with stories of suggestions being executed as though they were absolute imperatives. Whether in an entertainment setting or in a clinical setting, subjects were expected to obey without hesitation, and without using critical judgment, and they often did so.

Frankly, I do not know the extent of the influence that hypnotic suggestions can have. I suspect that in the right setting, the influence can be profound, yet published research neither confirms nor denies this. These questions are academic for me; they do not enter my practice. I am careful to frame the suggestions I give strictly as suggestions, thereby avoiding taking greater control of my patients. I urge all clinicians to do the same. It is true that, as the depth of trance increases, suggestions may be phrased more as directives without risking challenge by the subject; however, to do so prematurely will compromise rapport, and to do so at all will risk violation of the patient's free will.

Suggestions can be communicated verbally or nonverbally. They may be implicit in a situation or the product of imagination. They may be positive or negative in nature, and they may imply immediate or delayed execution. However, in all cases, suggestions must pass one test before integration: they must be accepted both consciously and unconsciously by the patient.

Pre-hypnotic suggestions are those suggestions offered before trance is experienced and are considered the most powerful of all suggestions.

Post-hypnotic suggestions are those offered during trance, to be executed after arousal from trance. That is, the "cue" for execution is to occur after arousal from trance.

Age Regression

"Age regression" and "regression" are terms found in many writings on hypnosis. The terms variously describe the use of enhanced memory capacity that is available in trance, and the use of trance to engender the "re-experience" of past events. It is my impression that most authors agree that the term only implies remembering, and this is how it is used in the present discussion.

Once an event is perceived, it is recorded in memory. This seems universally true at all ages. Unaided, conscious recall of an event may be inhibited or enhanced by many factors, including time, emotional involvement and reinforcement. However, discomforting or traumatic events tend to be the most difficult to recall. Recall of an event can also be blocked by a conscious belief that it cannot be remembered, or by an unconscious protective influence. Memory aided by hypnosis may not be effective in evading such blocks, depending upon many factors, including the responsiveness of the subject to hypnosis, the skill of the guide, and the severity of the experiences involved.

There is no informed disagreement with the contention that the trance state of hypnosis does enhance memory. Memory enhancement has been conclusively confirmed in many settings and contexts (see Chapter 4). The clinical value of such enhancement of memory is apparent. Significant elements that were responsible for lasting negative influence can be identified, and the issue resolved by exposure to more mature reasoning and understanding.

It is essential that anyone utilizing regressive phenomena exercise all possible precautions to avoid the "recall" of events that did not actually happen, events that are the product of the subject's imagination. The occurrence of such pseudo-memories can be avoided by careful wording of the suggestions used to elicit the memories. A clinician's suggestions should specifically relate to the objective of the search, avoiding implications for expected responses and avoiding any demand for response. As has been conclusively demonstrated by Pettinati (1988) and others, memories retrieved during the trance state tend to be strongly perceived by the subject as real and actual, sometimes in the face of evidence to the contrary. Such memories have the potential of serious consequences, both to the patient and to the therapist, if subsequently acted upon by the patient as though they are real and actual.

Age Progression

Accurate practice of any skill improves performance of that skill. It is no surprise that mentally rehearsing a behavior, an attitude, or a thought pattern, will improve these as well. Guiding a patient to mentally rehearse a behavior in desired ways provides the opportunity for practice. The advantage of doing so in trance lies in the ability we have of making it *real* – of making the experience so rich it's as though it's actually happening. Guiding the patient to incorporate all of the senses in creating the imagined, desirable situation facilitates making it subjectively real. Suggestions relating not only to sensitivity to visual experience, but also to sounds that might be associated with the situation, odors that might be present, tactile sensations, and even tastes might be appropriate. Since our imaginations truly do not know any limits, this process is easily engineered.

Guiding the patient to creatively imagine a situation never experienced, such as being competent in a new job, or functioning without the presence of a recently deceased loved one, provides opportunities for problem-solving and decision-making in a protected way. In this way a patient is able to anticipate problems.

Abreaction

The reader is referred to Chapter 5 for a discussion of this topic.

Time Compression and Expansion

Patients are commonly surprised by how quickly time passes while in trance. This happens spontaneously, and yet subjectively perceived time can also be altered by suggestion. While being guided to review a memory of some event, the patient may respond to a suggestion for the slow, detailed review of the memory. For example, *"The details will pass slowly in review, so you can be aware of each detail, and understand each detail, before the next detail comes forward in your memory."* Alternately, the suggestion for rapid review of many memories may be accommodated, as in, *"As I remain silent, permit an entire series of memories to pass in review, so that you can become aware of the relationship between them, and the effect they have had on you."* Or, as taught by Yapko (2003), *"Take a few moments, and those few moments will be all the time in the world you will need."*

Visualization

Some of us think visually – we "see" the spelling of words, we "see" the solutions to problems. Some argue that all of us have the ability to visualize; others will deny this is true. Perhaps it is simply a matter of semantics, in which the words have different meaning, or perhaps it is a matter of perception – how else could one person recognize another without some form of visual reference for comparison?

In any event, while in trance, almost everyone can create visual images in their mind's eye, and such images can provide solutions to problems, guidance toward goals, and insights into origins of dysfunction. The *inability* to visualize a given situation in a patient who is otherwise able to visualize can be informative in its own right, as it is likely an indication of unconscious blocking of that subject matter.

Desensitization

It is accepted that repeated exposure to a stimulus, while preventing response to it, will result in diminished response to that stimulus; we become progressively desensitized to it. This same diminished response is also created in trance work by means of direct suggestion, or by means of imagined, repetitious rehearsal of a stimulus void of a response.

Dissociation

Aspects of dissociation have been discussed in Chapter 3. As an overview, consider that when an anxious patient is being guided to experience trance, an immediate calming effect occurs that is evident to an observer, and is evident to the patient as well. The patient is *dissociated* from his or her emotions. The mental capability of removing ourselves from a situation, to "not think" about something, or to "not be aware" of something, is greatly enhanced by the use of trance.

In the clinical situation, dissociation is a very useful tool in work involving negative or uncomfortable emotions. Most patients in trance will spontaneously experience dissociation from emotional influence, that is, they will be capable of thinking about an emotion without subjectively experiencing that emotion. Moreover, even those patients who may spontaneously abreact to a particular event can be taught, by suggestion, to set the emotion "over there," and to continue to enjoy being comfortable, while doing the necessary intellectual work.

Techniques to Accomplish Insight

Spontaneous Awareness

A basic hypnotic technique can be to suggest to a patient in trance that there be spontaneous, conscious awareness of any purpose or function of the symptom being experienced. In many cases this can be the most expeditious. The greatest problem with this approach is that of differentiating between conscious thoughts and opinions, and the kind of spontaneous awareness that can come from the unconscious. In the end, the test of success is in the real world: Is the consciously desired change in effect now?

Free Association

Even without trance, the free association technique taught by Freud can be employed to reveal some psychodynamics of dysfunction. With trance, the technique is far more efficient.

Age Regression

The characteristic of trance that permits the subject to review an event that occurred in the past can be a powerful way to identify emotional roots and underpinnings of symptoms. Several hypnotic techniques are available to guide the patient to such roots, including the affect bridge, the memory bridge, the somatic bridge, and the time bridge. These are discussed in following paragraphs. In each of these techniques, the patient is guided to access memories by "bridging" back in time to a related memory.

In using the *Affect Bridge*, as taught by Watkins (1978), the suggestion given might be as follows:

> *As you review a recent memory of the problem, identify some feeling that is also present, a feeling that may be physical, emotional or a combination of both. Do you recognize what I'm talking about? Good. Now, let there be a memory of a not-so-recent time when you were feeling that particular way, when you were feeling that particular feeling. It might be just moments ago, or hours or days ago, but some recent time when that feeling was present. Let me know when that memory is present. Good. I'd like you to pay particular attention to that feeling, so you will recognize it if you experience it again. And now, I'd like you to carry that feeling back in time, to another place, another time, when that same feeling was present. It might have been long ago, or perhaps not so long ago. Another time, another place. And when that memory is there, I ask that you share it with me. Where were you? What was happening? Was that same feeling present?*

After eliciting the memory, examine it for the presence of the problem symptom and to recognize the association between the symptom and the emotional content. Then, earlier memories of the emotion can be sought by repeating the suggestion for bridging backwards, until no earlier memories are revealed. Suggestions similar to the following might be used:

> *Again, I ask that you bring that particular feeling (the bridge) to your mind. Perhaps remember the more recent time when it was present, and let me know when you have that feeling in mind. Good. Now, again, I'd like you to take that feeling back in time, to another place, another time,*

perhaps this time to the very first time you ever experienced that feeling. Now, what is there, where are you in this memory?

When the earliest memory has been elicited, and the relationship between the event and the symptom is clear to the patient in terms of current, more mature knowledge and understanding, guide the patient to consider the appropriateness of the influence of the event now, at this time in life. If the conclusion is negative, and if the relationship between the event and the symptom is understood, a simple, direct suggestion for relief will likely be effective, whereas before the regression it would not have had an impact.

In the case of the *Memory Bridge*, suggestion for the memory of a specific event is recommended. An example might be this suggestion: *"And now, as I touch your hand, be curious to see what memory comes to your mind. Let it be the memory of the first time you ever experienced that situation. Let the memory become sharp and clear, so that you understand what was happening, and the effect it had on you."*

In the case of the *Somatic Bridge*, suggestions for the memory of a particular physical sensation can be suggested. An example follows: *"And now, with the next breath you take, perhaps there will be a memory, a memory of the first time you ever experienced that particular physical sensation. If you are willing, share that memory with me."*

Examples of the use of the *Time Bridge* include: *"When I touch your hand, be curious to see where you are and what is happening in that memory. Let it be the third time you rode a bicycle. There may have been many times when you spoke harshly, and you can remember many of those times now, while I am silent."*

Ideomotor Questioning

The reader is referred to the work of Cheek (1994) for an exhaustive discussion of this subject. In employing this technique, responses from the unconscious are elicited and are communicated to consciousness by means of coded finger signals, which is Cheek's preferred mechanism, or by other motor mechanisms that can involve any muscle system of the body. The responses are involuntary; the responding finger lifts (often) to the surprise of the patient. Typically, the fingers are coded such that elevation of the index finger corresponds to a "yes" answer, the middle finger a "no" answer, the little finger means "I don't know," and the thumb means "I don't want to answer." In all events, answers are limited to those that have been coded, mandating a series of related questions to arrive at understanding of an issue.

In some situations, use of this technique is enhanced by the trance state; in others, trance seems unnecessary. It is the case, however, that in the course of employing the technique, spontaneous trance is commonly experienced. In any event, the unconscious mind of the patient is questioned about possible influences, unrecognized consciously, that may be exacerbating the problem in either duration or intensity. By this means, conscious insight may be obtained.

In their highly significant book, *Clinical Hypnotherapy*, Cheek and LeCron (1968) identified seven keys, or causative factors, that underlie psychosomatic illnesses. Appropriate use of these keys can speed the identification of causative factors by a process of elimination. This is especially true if the search for cause employs ideomotor questioning, since the answers are limited to "yes-no" or other simplistic responses. The keys identified by Cheek and LeCron follow:

1. *Conflict* Do the causal factors result from a desire to do something that is prevented by moral codes or societal taboos?

2. *Motivation* Does the symptom serve some purpose, such as protection, punishment or avoidance?

3. *Identification* Is the patient mimicking or otherwise copying another's behavior?

4. *Masochism* Is the symptom a form of self-punishment for some unconsciously perceived guilt that deserves punishment?

5. *Imprinting* Is there an idea that has become fixed in the unconscious domain, much as a post-hypnotic suggestion might become fixed?

6. *Organ language* Is the symptom a physical demonstration of expressions, such as, "That makes me sick" or "I can't swallow that," and "That gives me a pain in the neck."

7. *Past experiences* Is the symptom a product of past events not revealed by the above questioning?

Inner Advisor

After presenting the concept that we sometimes seem to have strengths, mental abilities, and wisdom that have gone unrecognized consciously, the suggestion that an Inner Advisor may exist is usually accepted at face value by patients; the consistency of responses subsequently obtained would advocate its validity. Furthermore, the suggestion that the patient listen to what that Advisor has to say usually elicits responses and cooperation from the Inner Advisor. Questions posed to the Inner Advisor can prompt responses that are surprising to both the patient and the therapist, and are often of marked therapeutic value. When posing questions to the Inner Advisor, address them to the Inner Advisor in the first person. For example, *"Inner Advisor, how old were you when ...?"*

Automatic Writing

Just as a subject in trance can perceive communications from the unconscious that are expressed by verbal statements (e.g., the Inner Advisor), or by coded physical motions (e.g., by ideomotor responses), expressions by writing may also be elicited. The subject in trance is given a pencil and paper, and placed in the position in which he or she would normally write, with the pencil posed above the paper. The suggestion is then offered that his or her unconscious can communicate by controlling the pencil, writing meaningful words on the paper. Specific requests may then be made and questions asked. As in the case of the Inner Advisor, responses obtained may require some interpretation and affirmation; however, they are apt to be both intelligent and informative.

Subliminal Therapy

The reader is referred to Chapter 12 for full description of this technique.

Chapter Five

Hypnotic Hypermnesia

Describing the relief from the horrific pain and terror,
And the consequent peace of mind,
Would be like a "newly sighted" person describing vision,
To a person who had never been blind.

Barbara Tierney, 2007

Hypermnesia, the recalling of memories not consciously accessible, is a subject of great controversy. Many people, some authorities included, maintain that these memories are often confabulated, and are always suspect. Lawsuits have been filed, books written, legislation created, and more than a few careers have been compromised as a consequence of memories of molestation and other offenses that were recalled while in trance. If exposed only to the information provided by the media, one might reasonably conclude that hypnosis is a menace to people. There are, of course, elements of truth in the claims and complaints, and there are also exaggerations and distortions. In this chapter, I defend the accuracy of events that are recalled when aided by hypnosis. The assumption that is in place is that the process of recall is conducted responsibly.

The highlight of many stage performances employing hypnosis is at the end, when the subject is guided to remember what he or she has just been doing. The reaction is usually hilarious and is a powerful demonstration of our capacity to selectively remember events, a capacity commonly demonstrated by forgetting unpleasant memories. Various explanations have been proposed to explain this inability to remember events that occurred during trance, but I have concluded that we simply do not know.

Amnesia may also result from direct suggestion; however, more elaborate approaches are usually indicated since the suggestion itself may be seen as a challenge to be defied. For example, the subject can be guided into trance while sitting facing a wall, guided to move to a different position during the trance experience, and then again be seated facing the original wall when roused from trance. The result will probably be amnesia for the trance experience. Unlike the entertainer, the therapist is apt to encourage memory of trance events. It is usually beneficial for the patient to remember, and the memory is easily elicited.

The phenomenon of trance amnesia that is responsible for the inability of a patient to consciously remember an event can also be responsible for a current dysfunction. It is as though trance had occurred incidentally at the time the dysfunction was learned, and the memory of the event is blocked by this spontaneous amnesia. For example, phobic persons are rarely able to remember how and when the phobia was learned. They may have a theory or two, and they may come close, but full comprehension of that initial, sensitizing event is not accessible without benefit of trance.

There may be questions regarding the factual accuracy of recalled events, and, while it is true that we have the capacity to creatively imagine "memories," the therapeutic benefits seem to accrue whether the memories are of actual or imagined events. However, in some situations, the issue of accuracy may be important and warrant further examination.

The fact that confabulation of hypnotically refreshed memory does occur, at least under some conditions, does not necessarily exclude accurate hypermnesia under other conditions. The emphasis on experimental research as the criterion for determining the accuracy of hypermnesia, when the validity of the experimental protocol is itself suspect in that the research was conducted using non-emotional content and academic subjects, may have led us astray in our evaluations. Various arguments are presented here in defense of the accuracy of hypermnesia inside and outside the courtroom.

By far the most convincing arguments questioning the veracity of hypnotically refreshed memory derive from the work of Helen Pettinati (1988). In her well-conducted research, she has convincingly demonstrated that not only can memories be confabulated while in trance; they also tend to be believed! This phenomenon is also evident in human behavior in other ways; however, it is particularly evident when a subject is in trance. There is a question of investigator bias in the design of her research; nevertheless, the results carry significant weight. Perhaps there is a real difference between results obtained when the data are derived from unemotional, staged reports, as compared to the reports clinicians receive about real-life events.

Nevertheless, *accurate* memories can be recalled, and hypnosis facilitates such memories. While the following considerations do not represent a comprehensive review of arguments for the accuracy of hypnotic hypermnesia, they do present a sampling of sufficient depth to defend it. They flag the need for examination of the question of accuracy from the perspective of *"accuracy"* as opposed to *"inaccuracy."* With responsible, informed guidance, it appears that recall under hypnosis actually avoids – rather than exacerbates – susceptibility to memory distortion, perhaps doing so by facilitating the bypass of barriers to memory, or by reducing anxiety and inhibition, or by increasing the susceptibility to suggestion for accuracy.

In this discussion, I will present the evidence for accuracy in decreasing order of persuasiveness, beginning with a brief discussion of controlled experiments having outcomes that substantiate accuracy, and ending with subjective arguments that appear to have some validity.

In Substantiation of Encoding All That is Perceived

Many have claimed that the mind records all perceived, meaningful information, whether perceived consciously or unconsciously, and that recall of such information is possible in a hypnotic trance. Although disputed, such claims are defensible in at least some respects.

Penfield (1975), in his classic studies of epileptic seizures, elicited spontaneous reports of earlier life experience by electrically stimulating specific locations in the brain, calling them "... electrical activations of the sequential record of consciousness, a record that had been laid down during the patient's earlier experience." He recounted, "I re-stimulated the same point thirty times (!), trying to mislead her, and dictated each to a stenographer. Each time I re-stimulated, she heard the melody again. It began at the same place and went on from chorus to verse. When she hummed an accompaniment to the music, the tempo was what would have been expected." Although the content of the memories elicited by Penfield was not statistically significant within the experimental situation, nor suggested by the operator (Penfield was "incredulous"), it was consistent with the concept of the encoding of all perceived information.

Chamberlain (1986; 1988), Cheek (1975), and Raikov (1980; 1982) present impressive evidence of the accurate recording of birth memories. This evidence includes the demonstration of non-volitional, physical patterns of behavior and of neurological reflexes and behavior, newborn reactions to stimulation, and of recalled events which occurred at the time of birth. These events were verified, in at least some instances. Hull (1933), in his classic work, referenced a variety of laboratory experiments that verified the efficacy of hypnotic hypermnesia.

Controlled Studies Positive for the Accuracy of Hypermnesia

Augustynek (1977) conducted a controlled experiment yielding positive evidence for the accuracy of hypnotically refreshed memory, even though the stimulus items were unrelated to the meaning of the recalled material.

Crawford and Allen (1983) demonstrated the efficacy of hypnosis in eliciting visual memory with intrinsic accuracy demonstrated by improved performance on tasks dependent on such memory.

In his study involving the recall of verse and prose learned at least one year previously, Strickler (1929) concluded that, "Hypermnesia in the trance state for sense material learned a year or more before has been clearly established." (108–119).

True (1949) questioned subjects about the day of the week of memorable dates, e.g., Christmas and birthdays, at ages four, ten and seventeen. Answers were compared to a perpetual calendar, and results showed 93% accuracy for tenth year, 82% accuracy for seventh year and 69% accuracy for the fourth year. These results would also logically correlate with subjects' age-sensitivity to, and perception of, dates and the days of the week.

White, Fox, and Harris (1940), in a well-designed study involving recall of poems learned over a year previously, demonstrated higher content accuracy of material recalled in hypnosis.

Comparisons of hypnotically obtained reports of mother and (now adult) child pairs by Chamberlain (1986) substantiated both the validity and accuracy of birth memories. Although inadequately controlled, this study utilized "dovetailing" of details in the reports, which occurred a total of 137 times, compared to a total of nine contradictions in the ten mother-child pairs examined.

Sears (1978) demonstrated enhanced recall using a visual display of easily recognized materials (e.g., penny, cup, camera), reporting "a consistent gain of hypnotic recall over waking recall." (296–304).

Studies Involving the Recall of Events that Occurred Under General Anesthesia

Studies conducted by Bennett (1988), Cheek (1975), and Erickson (1989a) confirm the phenomena of hypnotic recall of events as perceived by the patient while under general surgical anesthesia. Since the patients were under adequate anesthesia, and were unable to recall the material without hypnosis, one possible explanation is that the experience must have been unconsciously perceived at the time of encoding. These studies primarily involved the post-anesthetic recall of auditory communications, resulting in inferences regarding the potential impact of such perceptions on the well-being of the patient. The accuracy of recalled material was substantiated in all studies.

Reported Instances of Verification of Material Obtained in a Forensic Setting

In a courtroom, the issue of accuracy of hypnotically refreshed memory is fundamental to the question of admissibility of testimony derived from such refreshment. If hypnotically refreshed memories were not accurate in a high percentage of instances, their value in the world of criminal and forensic investigation would approach zero, and hypnosis has a well-documented history of success as an investigative tool. Moreover, as suggested by DePiano and Salzberg (1981), Dhanens and Lundy (1975) and Kroger and Douce (1979), hypnotically refreshed memories are likely to be more accurate and detailed than non-hypnotically refreshed memories.

In his penetrating evaluation and critique of studies of whether hypnotically refreshed memory should be allowed in courtroom testimony, Watkins (1989) concluded such testimony should be allowed:

> "Out of these claims and counter-claims, examinations and cross-examinations, the adversarial system will operate as it does in other areas," and "…we are not ready yet to conclude that hypnotic memory enhancement should 'never' be permitted in the courtroom and, hence, we should not at this time be initiating campaigns aimed at convincing courts to adopt such a position." (71–83).

Numerous reports point to forensically valuable information being obtained by hypnotically refreshed memory. Beyond the reports of non-sensational uses of hypnosis for investigative purposes by Reiser (1976), Reiser and Nielson (1980), Schafer and Rubio (1978), and others, there are the more sensational examples, such as the Chowchilla kidnapping in which the location of kidnapped children was located by hypnotically refreshed memory. This case was reported by Kroger and Douce (1979). Indeed, there seems to be little question of the value of hypnosis as an aid in criminal investigation. This is affirmed by the American Medical Association, Council on Scientific Affairs (1985) published position, and by Orne et al. (1984), in their published guidelines for the conduction of investigative interviews.

Reiser and Nielson's (1980) report states, "Of the information obtained with hypnosis where corroboration was possible, 90.7% was found to be accurate" (p. 184). This is particularly persuasive in making a case for the accuracy of hypermnesia, at least for meaningful material (as opposed to the non-sense material often employed in experimental studies), and perhaps for material recorded under stress.

Spanos et al. (1987), concluded that hypnotically obtained memories carry with them a subjective conviction of validity, and that hypnotically engendered pseudo-memories are no more resistant to cross-examination than are other memories:

> "Our findings provide no support for the notion that hypnotic interrogations facilitate the formation of pseudo-memories. Contrary to the implications of this hypothesis, hypnotic subjects were (a) as likely to be misled by a leading interrogation, and as likely to misidentify a suspect, as non-hypnotic subjects, (b) no more confident in their misidentifications than non-hypnotic subjects, and (c) at least as likely as non-hypnotic subjects to break down under cross-examination by disavowing their initial misattributions and their initial misidentifications." (pp. 271–89)

Studies Demonstrating the Phenomena of Abreaction with Restored Physiological Responses of an Earlier Period

In the usual clinical situation, we tend to consider memory as consisting of conscious recollection of material that was originally perceived via one or more of the senses. However, by expanding our concept of memory to include physiological responses encoded in infancy, without conscious awareness, distinct gauges of accuracy become apparent. Cheek (1975) related patterns of maladjustment, including physical maladjustment, to imprinting at birth. Erickson (1937) described the development of apparent unconsciousness during hypnotic reliving of a traumatic event in which unconsciousness was experienced. LeCron (1972) reported objective studies of eye-movement patterns, recovery of Babinski signs, and alteration of responses from plantar flexion to dorsiflexion, during abreaction of infancy.

Also, Raikov (1980) conducted a series of experiments in which newborn reactions obtained in hypnotic regression were compared with such reactions obtained by role-playing. The reactions obtained by aid of hypnosis were judged highly accurate, while those obtained by role-playing were judged highly inaccurate. Additionally, Raikov (1980) had trained neurologists to evaluate the neurological reflexes and behavior of subjects regressed to infancy with results "quite convincing" to them. Wolberg (1948) reported, "Some subjects can be regressed to the neonatal period, as demonstrated by sucking and grasping movements and an inability to speak while regressed" (43).

Reported Instances of Verification of Hypnotically Refreshed Memories

Although lacking the controls of academic research, clinicians typically and frequently report instances in which some significant item of information obtained during a clinical interview under hypnosis is confirmed by the patient via other sources of information. For example, "Mother told me that she *did* have long hair when I was that age." Repeated instances of such reports, coupled with the obvious benefits of employing hypnosis for therapeutic analysis, result in a subjective conclusion on the part of the clinician that such memory is accurate. To be sure, this conclusion may be biased in favor of accuracy by several factors, such as the need of the patient to be believed; nevertheless, the frequency of such experience must be weighed as significant.

Subjective Evidence Affirming the Accuracy of Hypnotically Refreshed Memory

In his teachings, Elman (1964) affirmed his conviction that memory under hypnosis is accurate, as have Erickson (1937; 1989a), LeCron (1965), Cheek (1975), Kroger (1976) and Kline (1955), in addition to many others. These "authorities" expressed opinions derived from the clinical, rather than the experimental situation. Frankel's (1988) comment that, "...the recall of meaningful, potentially emotion-laden, personal memories remains a clinical exercise that is not easily duplicated in a laboratory setting" (250) has particular relevance here.

Subjective reports are responsible for the initiation of virtually all psychological research. Moreover, we tend to pay attention to the subjective reports of those whom we respect. Consider the subjective reports of Cheek (1975), LeCron (1965), Erickson (1937), and Kroger (1976), and many others, all of whom consistently express the efficacy of hypnosis in psychotherapy, with at least a strong implication of both the existence and the accuracy of hypermnesia exhibited in the context of psychotherapy. Subjective reports are often discounted because of reported "research," even though the research is controversial, as in the case of hypnotic hypermnesia. It is perhaps unwise to arbitrarily discount such reports; surely the collective opinion of so many responsible clinicians should carry some weight.

It has been argued that the very suggestible status of the subject in hypnosis produces a situation in which iatrogenic influence can result in confabulation. Perhaps because of my consistent sensitivity to the issue, this claim has not been verified by my experience. In repeated, deliberate attempts to alter reported memory, I have consistently found subjects highly resistant to overt, and covert, suggestions that modify the details of any memory. That I may be unconsciously and covertly influencing subjects' memory is clearly possible, but I judge the possibility remote.

Studies Comparing Recall of Sense versus Non-sense Material

When doing research in the laboratory setting, we strive for objective measures of the variables we study. In doing so we sometimes unwittingly introduce extraneous variables that can compromise external validity. In studying memory, the researcher is tempted to employ non-sense measures, such as unrelated words or strings of numbers because they are more easily reduced to objective measures; however, doing so appears to contradict the results obtained when sense material is employed.

The literature demonstrating inaccuracy of hypnotically refreshed material does include reports of confabulation of sense material, yet most of the published evidence for inaccuracy involves non-sense measures. This is true in spite of the fact that comparisons of hypnotically recalled sense versus non-sense material consistently confirm significantly improved recall of the former, and lack of improvement of the latter. DePiano and Salzberg (1981), Dhanens and Lundy (1975), Erdelyi (1988), Frankel (1988), Rosenthal (1944), Shields and Knox (1986), Stager and Lundy (1985), Stalnaker and Riddle (1932), and White et al. (1940), all report this same theme, even though derived from varied approaches in researching the subject. Rosenthal (1944) and Pascal (1949) concluded that hypnosis enhanced recall, even of non-sense material, when the learning occurred under stress.

Spinhoven and Wijk (1992) examined age regression in both the experimental and the clinical setting, concluding both that, "Patients obtained significantly lower scores for experimental age regression than for clinical age regression, in particular when the experimental assessment preceded the clinical assessment of age regression," (43) and that "These findings give a tentative indication that more patients are able to experience clinical age regression than can be predicted from their responses to an experimental suggestion for hypnotic age regression, where almost no opportunities for patient contact or maximizing of hypnotic responsiveness are provided" (40).

***

It is clear to me that hypnosis facilitates *accuracy* of memory. This may be by reducing anxiety, releasing inhibition, or facilitating access to unconsciously stored material. Perhaps published emphasis on the *inaccuracy* of hypermnesia is misdirected and research emphasis should now be placed on identifying what is accurate, rather than on what is inaccurate.

It seems premature to exclude hypnotically refreshed memory from the courtroom. We need to know more about the mechanisms of memory encoding, accessing and retrieving before dispensing with its use. Cross-examination of witnesses has served us well in uncovering truth; it will serve the same purpose whether the testimony is or is not hypnotically refreshed. Moreover, the demonstrated value of the additional information available through the use of hypnosis, in combination with cross-examination, far outweighs any risk that might be incurred.

Part II

Clinical Considerations

Chapter Six

Two Basic Approaches to Using Hypnosis

There will come a time when you have to acknowledge
that your parents will never be the people you hoped they would be.

Gwen Yager, 1995

Hypnosis is used for many purposes: entertainment, religious, business, forensic, research, and clinical. The scope of this book is limited to the clinical uses of hypnosis, and within that domain there are two approaches: the use of direct suggestions, and the analytical use. In this chapter, the two are defined and delineated with respect to situations in which their use is appropriate. Understanding the two classifications will aid the clinician in choosing the most effective intervention.

The published literature on the application of hypnosis in relieving human suffering – physical and mental – is largely limited to its use in the context of the clinician making direct suggestions to the subject for the subject's well-being. Such use has merit in many situations. However, in situations where the effectiveness of such suggestions is inadequate, or where response to the suggestion is not forthcoming, the opportunity to utilize the characteristics of trance to uncover and resolve causal factors has been largely overlooked.

Clinically, the two methods for utilizing the phenomena seem evident and separate:

1. Hypnotic trance can be used as a state of mind in which suggestions of a "symptomatic" nature are offered; that is, suggestions that are oriented toward alteration of the symptom itself, as opposed to addressing causal factors, or toward exploring related material. Examples of this class of suggestion would

be, *"You will never again want to smoke,"* and, *"You will find you are free of the compulsion to scratch yourself."*

2. Trance can also be used as a vehicle of inquiry, of analysis, and as a means of reframing causal factors, thereby eliminating the undesired symptoms. This application may rely on the characteristic of enhanced memory capacity that is afforded by trance, or it may rely on spontaneous insight, gained without overt analysis. An example of such applications includes the recall of a memory of an initial sensitizing event responsible for a given (undesired) symptom, followed by exploration of reinforcing experiences, thereby discerning its etiology. From the position of understanding the etiology, reasoned judgment can be used to eliminate the conditioned response by maturely reaching conclusions contrary to the initial conclusion, thereby eliminating the symptoms.

Risks and advantages exist within both methods. If hypnosis is used only as a vehicle for suggestions for the relief of symptoms, the unresolved underlying influence of an unconscious nature may surface in the future, even though a favorable immediate response to the suggestion is obtained. While this approach can be time-efficient, there are many occasions when suggestions are not integrated beyond the immediate response. Then they are somehow eventually rejected by the patient, either consciously or unconsciously. The use of hypnosis as a tool for uncovering and resolving causal influence is an option in such situations, and may result in protracted relief or even "cure." On the other hand, if hypnosis is used only for analytical purposes, unnecessary time may be expended; symptomatic suggestion may have resolved the problem more economically.

In my practice, the flow of treatment between the two "methods" is sometimes difficult to separate. There have been some cases in which I used one or the other separately, but both are serially involved in most cases. It is my belief that essentially all of my patients can benefit from the skill of self-hypnosis. I therefore typically begin treatment by teaching that skill. The course of treatment from that point on is dependent upon the presenting problem, the patient's preference, and my clinical judgment regarding the goals.

I uphold Carl Rogers' position that the patient must be the center and focus of effective therapy.

As a simple example, if I am helping someone to stop smoking, I will first teach the person self-hypnosis. Then, depending upon my clinical judgment and the patient's wishes, I may utilize the suggestive approach without taking the time for analysis. I do this knowing the analytical approach can be used if the suggestive approach is not effective. I do this knowing that about one in four people will stop smoking on at least a semi-permanent basis with suggestions alone, and the additional expense of analytical work is not justified if this patient is one of those four. Similarly, when treating childhood asthma, I will only use the suggestive approach, unless it turns out to be insufficient. On the other hand, when treating asthma in an adult, I assume that secondary gain has accumulated and I will consistently use analysis.

Using Hypnosis as a Suggestive Vehicle

Historical Perspective

Throughout the history of hypnosis, clinicians have recognized that a subject in trance is more suggestible than when not in trance. Only in recent decades has its value as an analytic tool been recognized.

Suggestibility

The dictionary refers to "suggestibility" as being a state in which we are readily susceptible to being influenced by suggestion, of being mentally susceptible to the influence and opinions of others. That definition is adequate for understanding the particular aspect of the trance state in which unusual, perhaps unexpected and even beneficial, responses can be elicited. Yet, in hypnotic work, it is important to recognize that a subject is only *more* suggestible than in the waking state. He or she is not in a state of total subjugation.

Advantages

A primary advantage of trance lies in the immediate benefits to be obtained, especially when a patient is highly motivated to respond and is in the presence of authority (as self-perceived by the patient). A trained and gifted physician can blend "suggestions" into his or her interactions with a patient, for the patient's benefit, even without awareness of the intervention by the patient. Overt or implied suggestions for comfort, absence of anxiety, reduced blood loss, rapid healing, and many other benefits, may have impressive effect.

Another primary advantage of the "suggestive" approach lies in the cost and time-efficiency in those situations in which it is effective in accomplishing the desired change, without requiring analysis of the problem. For example, a patient demonstrating a compulsive behavior and who desires to stop the behavior can be offered suggestions in trance to the effect that he or she will "never behave that way again." As mentioned previously, case reviews indicate that in about one-in-four cases such suggestions are adequate for the purpose; the person stops the behavior for a prolonged period without difficulty. In the remaining three cases, analytical work is indicated.

Using Hypnosis as an Analytic Tool

Analysis, as used here, does not refer to Freudian psychoanalysis, even though hypnosis can be used to facilitate free association. Instead, it is goal-directed work, and the goal should be identified in advance of treatment, at least in a general sense. It is the uncovering of repressed material, thereby obtaining insight into current problems by identifying their unconscious roots. It is a matter of developing personal understanding of the etiology of problems, thereby enabling desired change by rational reinterpretation (reframing) of the causal influence.

Historical Perspective

Early proponents of the use of hypnosis for analytic purposes are exemplified by Wolberg (1945), Watkins (1949), Linder (1952) and Weitzenhoffer (1957). These clinicians maintained that for healing to take place it is necessary for the patient to *re-experience* early events – in other words, to experience abreaction – as opposed to simply *remembering* the events under hypnosis. More recently, therapists such as Cheek and LeCron (1968) have de-emphasized the necessity for abreaction, favoring instead the achievement of an intellectual, cognitive understanding of events. This is the perspective I endorse.

Concerns about Using Hypnosis Analytically

Spiegel (1997) and others, including Yapko (2003) in his discussion of the *Critical Incident Process*, have cautioned against the use of hypnosis to recover suppressed memories. Terms such as "hazardous" are used, based on concerns about re-traumatizing the patient by re-exposure to earlier trauma, or by overwhelming the ability of the patient to integrate the material that is uncovered.

I share the concern of my colleagues; however, I am far less concerned about the degree of risk. In treating many hundreds of patients, I have yet to encounter a situation where injury resulted from either regression to, or abreaction of, memories of traumatic events. Perhaps my expectation that the patient will benefit from the exploration, as opposed to risking injury, is responsible for the benefits achieved. Perhaps in those reported cases where injury resulted, it was due to the expectation of the therapist, which was covertly communicated to the patient, that harm might result.

When I interact with an emotionally charged patient who expresses concern about reviewing possibly traumatic memories, I will not pressure the patient to do such work. Yet, I will point out that, *"Whatever that event might have been, you survived it the first time and you can certainly survive the memory of the event now."* After further education about the potential benefits, and the protective process to be engaged, patients are usually reassured and express a desire to explore their history. We start with a pleasant memory, then one of minor trauma, and they are then open to the benefits of unrestricted exploration.

The Role of Hypnosis in Accomplishing Change

In my view of human experience, we are conditioned creatures. We are conditioned by heredity, life-experience, and by spiritual forces that are not well understood. If this view is accurate, it further implies that if conditioning by experience has occurred, reconditioning must be possible. If we learn a dysfunctional behavior or an irrational fear, it makes sense that it is possible to relearn that effect in a different way, with different consequences – assuming we know how to do so. Often, the problem is that knowledge of the etiology of the learned dysfunction is retained in the unconscious domain, impervious to conscious desire or will.

We may gain insight into a problem and/or its origin by many means, including free association, dream analysis, and hypnotic age regression. However, insight alone is of little value in bringing about change. Another step is required, the step of intellectual understanding of cause, coupled with an intellectual decision/ conclusion/commitment to change based on that understanding.

The steps of resolving causal influence are straightforward: First, there is the requirement for insight about the etiology of the problem. Direct hypnotic suggestions for memory of precipitating events are often effective in accomplishing this step. Second, reasonably comprehensive, conscious understanding of the process whereby the original conditioning occurred must be achieved. This understanding must be achieved from the perspective of present, more mature knowledge about self and life, as contrasted with the limited understanding that was in effect at the time the precipitating event/s occurred. Third, on the basis of the new understanding obtained, the individual must make an intellectual decision about the appropriateness and advisability of the earlier influence continuing in present life. It seems the structured, cognitive recognition that the influence is inappropriate is essential to change; recognition of causal influence alone is not sufficient.

The Advantages of Using Trance in Analysis

Protection by dissociation. Hypnotic trance is defined as a dissociative experience. One advantage of this phenomenon is that, with appropriate guidance, the patient can dissociate from the emotional content of a memory, thereby permitting intellectual consideration without distress. A frequently encountered barrier to age-regression is the conscious fear of re-experiencing the trauma of an event, a fear that is often encountered, even when the patient is unable to articulate its basis. Reassurance may take the form of words such as: *"It is only necessary that you remember the event. It is not necessary that you re-experience what happened back then. Just as you can remember what you had for breakfast this morning, even though you are not having that breakfast now, you can remember what happened back then without experiencing the emotions you experienced then, remembering without distress."*

Enhanced recall. Although the issues of accuracy and the validity of hypnotically refreshed memories are debated, where clinical work is concerned it may not matter whether or not a memory is accurate in an absolute sense. Perhaps, if the recovered material is sufficiently real to the patient, it can be utilized to effect desired change despite inaccuracies. If a patient in trance recalls being locked in a dark closet and feeling terrified, and is thereby able to understand the genesis of a current fear of the dark, and to then eliminate the phobia, what does it matter if the memory is accurate?

The clinician is urged never to validate any reported memory, or to provoke memories by leading suggestions of content. However, this is not to say the clinician should avoid using responsible uncovering techniques. The likely benefits are far too great to abandon their use. Rather, the clinician is advised to proceed with the caution that comes with adequate training and experience, seeking corroborating information where appropriate.

Enhanced objectivity. Our ability to think objectively about an issue is consistently jeopardized by emotional experience. When we are angry, or afraid, or grief stricken, or are in the throes of various other emotions, our judgment is compromised. In trance, with the accompanying dissociation from emotion, we are better able to be objective in our understanding and analysis of undesired influence.

Compliant response. Every clinician has encountered the patient who does not comply with treatment, or who is so self-absorbed and verbose that the course of therapy is interrupted. When guided into trance, such patients spontaneously demonstrate an absence of volitional activity. Thus, they become silent and open to concepts presented by the therapist. Additionally, they are considerably more receptive to the assignment of tasks to be performed outside of the therapy session.

Chapter Seven

The Roles of Hypnosis in Psychotherapy

New Perceptions, feeling, and desires,
As I incrementally become awake,
From a slumber I engaged in,
Initially for survival sake.

Barbara Tierney, 2006

Hypnosis is being employed with increasing success as a clinical intervention in medicine and psychology. Yet the roles of hypnosis differ among the disciplines in terms of both technique and purpose. Although this book addresses procedures and applications in general, this chapter focuses on the discipline of psychology, addressing the classes of disorders in which hypnosis is either the treatment of choice, or is indicated as an adjunctive treatment. Hypnosis is, of course, but one of many treatment choices. Nevertheless, where appropriate it is the most effective intervention available, and should be considered in all cases.

Relieving Psychic Distress

Whether depressed, anxious, or experiencing another ego-dystonic state of mind, patients have probably become obsessed with their experience and may have difficulty relating to any other reality. In this situation, *properly* guiding the patient to experience the trance state will likely afford immediate symptomatic relief and act as an anchor for further work. Since any emotion may be either relieved or intensified in the trance state, "properly" means taking care to guide the patient's thinking *away from* the obsession. For example, in working with a depressed patient, after achievement of the trance state, suggestions – both specific and implied – must be offered for awareness of aspects of life that he or she *can* control (Yapko, 1992). As another example, when working to achieve relief

71

from pain, suggestions should be made to guide the patient to focus on a pain-free location. Any suggestions to the contrary – or simply the absence of suggestions – are apt to exacerbate the experience. (In this example, it should be noted that cause is not considered. Only the symptoms are addressed with the patient being guided by suggestion to awareness of only desired sensation, experience, and abilities. Further analytic work to identify and resolve causal influences may or may not be indicated.)

In some instances, patients may respond adequately to "symptomatic" suggestions, as above, making further treatment unnecessary. Frequently, however, even in those instances where relief is immediate, total, and dramatic, the symptoms are apt to return within minutes or days of arousal from the trance state. In such instances, long-term relief will likely require identification and resolution of unrecognized causal factors. When this is the case, after induction of trance, the patient would be guided to take advantage of expedited access to pertinent memories to uncover the cause and resolve that influence.

Although satisfying explanations for the mechanism of enhanced recall ability in trance are lacking, the reality of such recall is well established (see Chapter 4). Although the accuracy of such memory may be challenged (just as with all human memory), the material elicited will likely be therapeutically beneficial. Moreover, the use of age regression and abreaction is not limited to searching for negative influence; memory is the repository of *positive* experiences and influences as well. A recalled series of experiences of success may be reaffirming, contradicting and counterbalancing a sense of helplessness.

Relief from physical and psychological distress may be obtained pharmacologically, after allowing time for absorption and distribution of the agent within the body. In the meantime, hypnosis may offer immediate relief, requiring only direct suggestions in trance. It is also true that, because of the compromised intellectual capacity and judgment that are often present with emotional disorders, medications may be necessary to permit psychotherapy to proceed at all. As mentioned previously, the trance state can provide protection from unwelcome emotional influence, and achievement of the trance state is a skill that can be learned, at least to some level of proficiency, by essentially everyone.

Resolving the Influence of Prior Trauma

Conditioned responses incident to trauma may persist for a lifetime. Phobias, tics, stuttering, compulsions, obsessions, sexual dysfunction and various psychogenic illnesses are all examples. It is as though a lesson learned in the initial sensitizing situation, a lesson that was clearly appropriate for that situation, continues to be controlling in spite of conscious rational recognition of its current inappropriateness. This theme, of course, is encountered countless times in our practices. A complicating treatment factor is that it also seems true that the traumatic nature of the initial experience may result in its memory being repressed, thereby making resolution difficult. In a variation on this theme, even if the patient does have conscious memory of the event, the patient may not be willing to think about or discuss it, unless offered the emotional protection afforded by hypnosis.

Thus, the use of the trance state, with its inherent capacity to permit dissociation from emotion, may permit therapeutically necessary recall and/or make it possible for the patient to confront and resolve the influence of an event. Reassuring the patient that only the memory of the sensitizing event is required, and that re-experiencing it will not be necessary, can mean the difference between resistance to therapy and satisfactory progress. One possibility is that the mechanism of enhancement of hypnotically refreshed memory is simply that of setting aside fears of recall. In any event, the use of the trance state can greatly enhance the course of therapy, both in terms of efficiency and thoroughness.

The concept of "resolving" influences from past experience is fundamental to analytic psychotherapy. Accomplishing this first involves the identification of causal influence, beginning with the initial sensitizing event, and including subsequent contributing events. Identification is followed by objective evaluation of these influences and events from the perspective of current, more mature knowledge and understanding. In understanding the etiology differently (i.e., from the perspective of current knowledge), the influence of that event in present life is altered in favorable ways. The trance state can dramatically facilitate this process. Finally, the appropriateness of the influence of the event in current life is evaluated and conclusions are reached.

Either dissociated memory or abreaction of a prior precipitating event is possible in the trance state, influenced by a cue as subtle as the tense of the verbs used in the process of guiding the patient to the memory. In therapy, the choice of dissociated memory versus abreaction rests largely with the therapist, based on clinical judgment of the moment. However, spontaneous abreaction does occur and must be appropriately managed in the best interest of the patient. Possibly the most effective means of orienting and anchoring the patient to the present, thereby avoiding abreaction, is by means of a gentle touch on the back of a hand, or perhaps placing a hand on the patient's forearm, coupled with a suggestion for orientation to the present such as, *"You are here with me, in this room, and as you feel the touch of my hand, you will know you are here, with me, and not in that past situation."*

In my opinion, the premeditated use of abreaction is seldom indicated and, in fact, is generally contraindicated by two factors: (1) because the very threat of "reliving" an experience can dissuade a patient from participating in the therapy at all, and (2) because of the time-consuming process of re-experiencing the event in real time. Reassurance that, *"It is not necessary that you re-experience that event; it is only necessary that you remember it – much as you might remember what you had for breakfast this morning,"* can open doors otherwise closed to therapy.

Behavior Modification

Behavior resulting from conditioned response can be altered in a number of ways, including:

- Avoidance techniques
- Flooding techniques
- Progressive desensitization
- Opposing responses that can be practiced until the dysfunctional conditioning is undermined or overwhelmed.

In each of these techniques, the hypnotic trance can be of great support (Kroger, 1976). Indeed, the trance state can facilitate each of them to a degree that is often surprising, both to the clinician and to the patient. The additional, adjunctive use of hypnosis to gain knowledge and understanding of the initial, sensitizing event, thereby permitting cognitive reevaluation of its elements, can prevail in the most resistant situations.

Altering Physiological Responses

The link between emotion and physiological response to that emotion has been well established (Cannon, 1953). Lists of physical changes that take place in response to various emotions have been compiled. Such lists include changes in vital functions, glandular function, blood chemistry, brain function, and the pattern of blood flow in the body.

Bodily functioning such as digestion, regulation of the pattern of blood flow within the body, respiration, and so forth, mediated largely by smooth muscle, takes place in controlled, "intelligent" ways that are specifically directed by the unconscious domain of the mind via the autonomic nervous system. Clearly, such functioning is not controlled at a conscious level of awareness. And, just as clearly, such functioning is indicative of a high order of unconscious intelligence. The correlations frequently observed between emotional state and physical disorders, such as asthma and tension headaches, as well as situational reactions such as inappropriate anxiety and many other psychogenic disorders, are common examples of the influence of unconscious intelligence that is misguided by unfortunate past experience.

In response to hypnotic suggestions, medical wonders such as anesthesia, limiting blood loss in surgery, cardio-conversion, moderated pain in childbirth and altered physiological response to medications, are routinely reported by those who premeditatedly employ hypnosis in their practice. The reader is referred to the work of Cheek (1975) and the lectures of Dr. Steve Bierman, for more information.

Wolf (1950), at one time a guiding authority in pharmacology, published a well-controlled landmark study of the effects of various chemical agents on the body, coupling the administration of the studied agents with suggestions for effects. Of the three agents studied, the one that was most sensational was the use of ipecac. In this study, ipecac was used as a *soothing* agent! Ipecac is the emetic that is typically administered in emergency rooms to induce vomiting and its effects are both immediate and dramatic to observe; one should never stand in front of a patient being given ipecac! Although Wolf did not use the word "hypnosis" in his publication, all of the prerequisites for trance were incorporated in his protocol. This study is a classic in the literature demonstrating the authority of mind over physiology.

***

The helping professions are missing a valuable, potentially helpful and economically advantageous modality of treatment when they ignore hypnosis. Its application in each of the areas described offers improved efficiency, flexibility and personal satisfaction for therapists and patients alike. Moreover, hypnosis can bypass resistance and engage abilities not otherwise available to the patient. Fortunately, training in the clinical use of hypnosis is now offered, at least on an elective basis, in most medical and psychological curricula.

Chapter Eight

The Risks of Employing Hypnosis

An altered state is like fertile soil.
We can produce healthy seeds to grown into healthy fruit-producing plants,
We can let the weeds overrun it,
Or we can let erosion wash it away in the storm.

Judith Acosta and Judith Simon Prager (2002)
The Worst Is Over

In some circles, hypnosis has a bad reputation. There have been various claims of negative consequences. However, those who are informed of its true nature have minimal concerns about its use, as long as it is employed responsibly by clinicians who have been adequately trained. Such training is available privately, as well as through workshops of *The American Society of Clinical Hypnosis* (ASCH), *The Society for Clinical and Experimental Hypnosis* (SCEH), and local divisions of these societies. Of course, risks are involved when hypnosis is utilized improperly or carelessly. However, those risks are minimized when it is conscientiously used. In this chapter, I provide an assessment of the risks, limiting my assessment to the clinical application of hypnosis.

The literature on hypnosis contains references to the so-called "dangers" of utilizing hypnosis, but they are surprisingly few in number. Some refer to risks of mental distress or impairment; others refer to risks of physical injury of one kind or another. In reviewing this literature, and in discussions with colleagues, I have defined four areas that encompass all of the specific, significant dangers mentioned. I detail these four areas in the sections that follow, with the caveat that in 40 years of practice I have not encountered even one of them at a serious level. Responsibly used, hypnosis is far safer than other interventions.

Masking Organically Based, Non-Psychogenic, Physical Symptoms

The many reports of the effective use of hypnosis as an anesthetic in birthing and in surgical procedures (see Chapter 5) become striking evidence of our mental capacity to alter perception. By suggestion, deliberate or unintentional, an individual in trance can be guided to be unaware of or not bothered by physical stimulation of any sort. However when such physical stimulation constitutes a symptom of organic illness, and that symptom is masked, the potential of harm to the patient becomes real.

Although most human pain is often exacerbated by emotion or other mental states, and may be entirely psychogenic, some causes of pain justify medical treatment. Therefore, the responsible mental health clinician must use care in differentiating between psychogenic and organically based pain. When in doubt, evaluation by a physician is indicated. Yet, there are clear indicators of psychogenesis. If the discomfort is cyclic, or correlated with specific situations or mental states, it is likely to be either psychogenic or, at the very least, emotion is a highly significant contributor to the problem. To illustrate, a person with a toothache can be successfully guided to be indifferent to that discomfort, provided there is a plan of action to correct the problem such as an appointment with a dentist. If that appointment is not kept, the toothache will likely reappear in force. On the other hand, if the pain of an impending rupture of the appendix can be masked, the consequence can be fatal, illustrating the importance of accurate diagnosis.

Creating or Exacerbating Anxiety

The characteristics of hypnotic trance are diametrically opposite to the symptoms of anxiety. Yet, occasionally, a patient in trance may spontaneously begin to demonstrate symptoms of anxiety, doing so without apparent provocation. Such response may be due to abreaction of a distressing event that has not been shared with the therapist, or may be due to unconscious thought processes. In either event, it is the responsibility of the clinician to guide the patient to relieve the symptoms and this is typically best accomplished by orienting the patient to the present, non-threatening situation. The use of touch is encouraged in this instance. With permission, the therapist should touch the patient's hand in a supportive manner and offer suggestions for awareness of the present, anchored by that touch, and reassurance that, *"You can feel my touch and be aware that you are here, in this place, with me, and whatever that distressing thought may have been, it is only a memory now, and it's okay to remember things without re-experiencing them."*

Exceeding Mental or Physical Limits

One of the more popular demonstrations of hypnosis employed by stage hypnotists is to select a petite woman from the demonstration group, guide her to achieve a state of physical rigidity throughout her body, position her suspended between two chairs, and then stand on her. Such demonstrations are impressive and, I can't help but believe, dangerous. There are limits to the strength of muscle and tissue, and a 250-pound man standing on a 100-pound woman in that situation must certainly approach such limits. Yet, I have interviewed several women days after their experience, and the worst consequence reported was a slight soreness of muscles. Actually, this phenomenon is practiced in the martial art Aikido as well, so perhaps my concern in this instance is misguided.

Clinicians are advised to carefully avoid offering suggestions for mental, or physical, performance that is beyond the capacity of the patient. Suggestions that are out of sync with a patient's tolerance are likely to lead to headaches or emotional reactions of anxiety or depression, at the very least. The ability to assess the variables comes with skill and experience.

Prompting False Memories

Our age of litigiousness has resulted in yet another "danger" of the use of hypnosis: prompting memories that are subjectively perceived as valid by the patient, yet have no bases in reality. The reader is referred to Chapter 4 for elaboration on this topic.

Research on the Risk of Using Hypnosis

Since a comprehensive review of all publications relative to the risks of the use of hypnosis is not reasonably achievable, a review of the articles published in the *Journal of the American Society of Clinical Hypnosis* was completed with the results presented in following paragraphs.

The Journal has been published quarterly since the formation of the Society in 1955. At least 1,000 articles have been published since then, with only eight of the articles addressing the risks of using hypnosis. These articles are listed below. Within these eight articles, 25 cases were described in sufficient detail for inclusion in this review and the results are tabulated as follows:

Cases of adverse consequences associated with the use of hypnosis

	By trained professionals — Total cases – 15															By non-professionals — Total cases – 10									
Nature of the consequence																									
Psychological	•	•	•		•	•	•		•	•	•		•	•	•	•		•	•	•	•				
Physical				•	•			•				•	•					•		•					
Behavioral																	•							•	•
Severity of the consequence																									
Severe	•				•	•		•					•			•			•	•	•	•			•
Mild		•	•	•			•		•	•	•	•	•			•	•						•	•	
Duration of the consequence																									
Long-term					•	•		•								•				•	•	•			
Short-term	•	•	•	•			•		•		•		•	•	•			•	•				•	•	•
Unreported										•		•				•									

The classification of the severity of the consequences was by subjective judgment on my part, and the classifications of "long-term" duration is defined as lasting for more than 24 hours, with "short-term" as lasting for less than 24 hours.

Included articles from the Journal of ASCH
Echterling, Lennis G. and Emmerling, David A., *Impact of Stage Hypnosis*. Vol. 29, No. 3, January 1987.

Klienhauz, M., Dreyfuss, D.A., Beran, B., and Azikri, D., *Some After-Effects of Stage Hypnosis: A case study of Psychotic Manifestations.* International Journal of Clinical and Experimental Hypnosis, 1979.

Mears, Ainslie, *An Evaluation of the Dangers of Medical Hypnosis.* Vol. 4, No. 2, October 1961.

Klienhauz, Moris and Beran, Barbara, *Misuse of Hypnosis.* Vol. 26, No. 4, April 1984.

Kleinhauz, Moris and Eli, Ilana, *Potential Deleterious Effect of Hypnosis in the Clinical Setting.* Vol. 29, No. 3, January 1987.

MacHovec, Frank, *Hypnosis Complication: Six Cases, Risk Factors, and Prevention.* Vol. 31, No. 1, July 1988.

MacHovec, Frank J. and Oster, Mark I., *In the Best of Families: Understanding Hypnosis Complications in Graduate and Post-Graduate Training Experiences.* Vol. 42, No. 1, July 1999.

MacHovec, Michael A., *Complications Following Hypnosis in a Psychotic Patient With Sexual Dysfunction Treated by a Lay Hypnotist.* Vol. 29, No. 3, January 1987.

***

Since all of the 25 cases reported involved hypnosis being employed in treating presenting disorders, it is not clear whether the consequences were caused by the hypnotic intervention, *per se*, were exacerbated by the hypnotic treatment, or were correlated with other undefined variables. However, considering that many of the 1,000 articles reported included multiple cases, the data suggest that less than one percent of all cases resulted in reported adverse effects of any kind, and many fewer cases involved serious consequences. As I stated previously: responsibly used, hypnosis is far safer than other interventions.

Chapter Nine

*The Significance of Hypnosis in Informed Consent**

*The body cannot tell the difference
between events that are actual threats to survival
and events that are present in thought alone.*

Joan Borysenko, Ph.D.

*My colleague, Steve Bierman, M.D., has lectured extensively on the
subject of hypnosis in the medical setting. In 1998 Dr. Bierman ended a
15-year career as an emergency room doctor. He was featured on the* CBS
News America Tonight *and* Dateline NBC, *and he lectures annually
to my classes in hypnosis at the UCSD School of Medicine, in addition to
offering his own courses. In the role of emergency doctor he made extensive use of hypnosis on a routine basis, pioneering such applications as
correcting cardiac arrhythmias and restoring joint dislocations without
manipulation. I have long considered his concepts concerning the hazards
of informed consent to be of great importance to all in the helping professions, and the reader is encouraged to consider this chapter seriously; it is
a transcription of one of his lectures.*

*Informed consent is mandated by federal and state laws. Patients are
legally entitled to information about the details and consequences of every
procedure prior to authorizing it. There is, however, the inherent risk of
negatively influencing the outcome by the use of ill-advised language in
communicating the information. In situations in which informed consent
is required, the patient is commonly in a state of mind that would be
identified as trance, even though no formal induction has been employed.
The choice of words and statements, as well as how they are presented,
becomes important because the content may be integrated as hypnotic
suggestions whether correctly understood or not. The following lecture by
Doctor Bierman presents the problem and its solution.*

---

* A lecture by Steven F. Bierman, M.D. to an advanced hypnosis class at the
UCSD School of Medicine, March 2001. Transcribed and presented here with
Dr. Bierman's permission.

Now that we understand how words affect clinical outcomes, words delivered with the hypnotic authority all clinicians possess, the questions come, "How do we deliver the inevitable bad news healthcare sometimes requires without having a deleterious effect on our patients?" and "How do we warn our patients of potential adverse side effects of drugs or procedures without harming them?" That is, "How do we explain a disease condition without worsening it?"

These are especially pertinent questions today, when clinicians are required to give informed consent to patients – to explain the pros and cons of a proposed treatment. So let's use informed consent as a model for how to deliver potentially damaging information.

To do this we will use three skills: anchoring, analogue marking and the use of the so-called general referential index. I will elaborate on these skills in a moment.

First, I will talk about the three components of every patient-doctor encounter: (1) information gathering, (2) synthesis/diagnosis and (3) information delivery (treatment/prognosis). The first two are what you learn in medical school; they are expected by the patient. So, when you make your "gold star" diagnosis, and somebody has some rare disorder you just read about in the *New England Journal* last week, and they walk into your office and you nail it, no one is going to say, "Great diagnosis, that's awesome." The patient expects that level of competence. In Part 1, you're going to get the patient's history and physical, various labs, X-rays, imaging and so forth. Then, in Part 2, you're going to learn how this makes sense, and to form, if possible, a single diagnosis to explain this spectrum of phenomena.

The patient will assume you know what you are doing and are perfect at it. If you aren't perfect at it, the patient will damn you for your inhumanity, your imperfection. The part they care most about is Part 3, information delivery. In the information delivery part of your encounter with the patient, you're going to tell them their diagnosis – what you think they have – and you're going to give them a treatment regimen, that is, what you think will work to make them better. Then you're going to give them, in some way, a prognosis. It might be anything from, *"I don't know how long it will* take for you to get well," to "Call me tomorrow, let me know how well you feel," to the full range in between. Hopefully, you will never say, "This is going to kill you," because if you diagnose someone with advanced pancreatic cancer today, you have no way of knowing they won't get killed by a Mac truck when they walk across the street, and the cancer has nothing to do with it. Hopefully, you won't prognosticate something with negative outcomes. Not that you won't be honest with someone and say, "Let's face it, this is a disease that kills people," but what I don't want you to say is, "You've got two months to live," because, I'll tell you right now, you don't know that! For every time you think you know a predictable outcome, there are exceptions. People with the exact same diagnosis have lived 10 to 20 times longer than others, and usually there is somebody who has survived the condition entirely. At least one person has survived and overcome almost everything, including juvenile onset diabetes, neuroblastoma, you name it.

When you get to the information delivery portion, you are going to offer a treatment plan. Also, you are required to *offer* informed consent; you are *not required* to give it if it is waived by the patient. Hear me again on this point; you are *required* to *offer* informed consent. That is what this lecture is about, not just about informed consent for hypnosis, but informed consent for any kind of treatment, or surgery, or manipulation of something. How you do that is *exceedingly* important.

There have been experiments showing that when you offer a negative suggestion, you get a negative outcome. If you tell people they will lose their hair, they will lose their hair. If you tell them they won't get well for three to five days, they won't. And, if you tell them they will be well in two-to-three days, they often are. How you deliver informed consent can color the clinical outcome. I want to spend some time giving you ideas on how to do this, because you're going to use this every day. In any given day, you're seeing 20 patients, and somewhere or other, in each case, you're required to give informed consent. It doesn't mean you will do it. You'll slip, you'll forget, you'll blow it off, or they'll waive it, but frequently you have to do it.

Here's a further example of the power and potency of your words as a physician: I had a patient who went in for spinal surgery with a doc, whom I personally believe is a poor technician, and who has very bad outcomes when he does spinal surgery. The patient came to me and said, "I want pre-op hypnosis for this," and I said, "Well, let's get specific, what is your primary issue?" Her primary issue was that she has been through multiple spinal surgeries in the past and she was phobic of hospitals, and could not get through the door. She knew she would pass out on her way to the door, and she wasn't going to make it in, and wasn't going to get the surgery. She wanted the surgery, and she had good rapport with this doctor and felt he was great (because *he* felt that he was great and she bought into that). It wasn't something I was going to interrupt, or something to interfere with.

So what is your *real* goal? "I want to get through the door and get in surgery, and get the IV (she had a phobia about needles as well) and have a good outcome." Okay, but what is your major focus in that? "The first two. Get me through the door and get the IV in. This other doctor can take care of it from there."

I had given her a host of suggestions (I worked with her three times) to get her into the hospital and through the door. It was a very positive outcome, and she went into the hospital eagerly, accepted her IV hungrily, and lay down with great expectations. Everything seemed just right. They had gotten into surgery, and I had given her all kinds of suggestions for post-op comfort, rapid wound healing, keeping your own blood, and all that. In surgery, they ran into some significant bleeding problems, and I would maintain that was because this particular surgeon often runs into bleeding problems. He is an orthopedic surgeon, doing complex spinal surgery. She came out of surgery and, while she was in the recovery room, she was comfortable, just waking up, the bleeding matters had been fixed, and she was offered patient-control anesthesia. She said she really didn't need it, and felt good.

When they were getting ready to transfer her, the surgeon came in and said, "Doctor Bierman must have given you the wrong suggestions because you bled like crazy in the operating room." Immediately, she had this terrible pain reaction, her blood pressure and pulse went sky high, they had to medicate her with intravenous morphine, and her whole post-operative course was a disaster.

Every time I have said to someone, as an Emergency Physician, to "normalize their heart," or "let their bones go back to an anatomic position"; every time I uttered a suggestion, I got a clinical response from it. That's my background and the source of my understanding of the belief that words matter. In this whole business of informed consent, that understanding of human response is the underpinning for me. It's why I'm so careful how I give it.

Most doctors believe they are obligated under the law to deliver informed consent to patients, whether they want it or not. Not true. You are obligated to *offer* such information. However, the patient has the right – and will often exercise that right if given the choice – to waive informed consent. Many patients, sensing at some level the potential harm such a communication may convey, simply do not want to hear what can go wrong with a procedure they are likely to undergo. "No thanks, Doc," they will often say, "I trust you... let's just get on with it." Should this be the case, your only obligation is to record in the chart: "Informed consent explained and offered, and expressly declined by patient." Remember this: A waiver of informed consent obviates the potential of misspeaking – which we are all prone to do. Patients know this and will regularly take measures to shut us up.

Let's assume that you believe, after you've done your H & P (History and Physical exam), and you've done, let's say, pelvic ultrasound, and they've got a suggestive shadow for appendicitis, and your diagnosis is *surgical abdomen to rule out acute appendicitis*. You go up to this patient and one of the first things, after you've delivered the diagnosis, is going to be the task of the physician, according to law, to relate all the risks and all of the benefits of surgery to the patient.

Remember the distinction in the language of hypnosis between a specific referential index, "you," and a general referential index such as "some people" or "Some patients I've known." That is a very, very key distinction; that is what distinguishes a doctor with hypnotic skills from someone who is klutzy with words. *"I am required by law to offer you information about the risks and the benefits that some people might experience from the surgery I am going to propose...."* You can hear how hypnotic language leaks in, even in simple expressions like that. *"But I am only required to offer it to you.*

If you prefer not to hear it, and simply go ahead with my advice, and go into the surgical procedure, that's fine too. I just need it to be clear that I'm offering the information, and if you want to hear it, I will happily provide it to you." Then they say, "You know what Doc," and I've heard this so many times, every day, especially from old-timers, "If you think it's the right thing to do, let's go for it, let's get this done."

"You sure you don't want to hear it?" "No, I don't. I don't want to hear it, don't want to think about it." You write in the chart, "Patient offered informed consent and expressly waived." This is a key point, because this gives your patient control over what they are going to hear.

Now, let's clarify those three terms I mentioned in the beginning. First, *anchoring*. This technique makes use of what psychologists call state-dependent learning. A man who learns to solve math problems with a pencil in his hand is more likely to solve a given problem when he, in fact, has a pencil in hand. A philosopher who learns to think abstractly with a pipe in his mouth is best at philosophizing later in life with a pipe in his mouth. And so on. Cues of various sorts – tactile, auditory, olfactory, topographical – become associated with something and so call to mind their associated part. Think, for example, of the smell of Grandma's house, or of fresh-cut grass – and you will call to mind a host of associated memories. In delivering information to patients, it will be useful to define a special area, which denotes "certainty" and another which denotes "uncertainty." Generally, the "certainty" area is, say, one small step toward the patient; the "uncertainty" area is one small step to the side. I'll show you shortly how and when to do this.

Next, *analogue marking*. Simply put, this technique is a way of underscoring, of marking, an idea so as to impart significance to it. Any discernible signal can be used for this purpose. For example, "There are some things that are – (hard clearing of the throat) – patently untrue." Here, the hard clearing of the throat is associated with things patently untrue. Next, you say, "Nixon was really a (hard clearing of the throat) good man." Believe me, your listener will get the drift. Analogue marking can be done, as I've just indicated, with certain vocal cues; but it can also be done with hand signals, distinctive breathing patterns, or any number of other distinctive behaviors.

Finally, as we warm up each section of the orchestra for a symphony of significant communications to our patients, there is the *General Referential Index*. This fancy term is best understood in contradistinction to the specific referential index "You." General referential indices are terms like: people, patients, someone. When you use such a term, the patient has the option to attach personal significance to the communication or not: *"I've had some patients who simply got better on their own in a matter of days...."*

We are going to use these three mechanisms to structure a communication to our patients that, while impeccably honest and accurate, imparts hope and may even predispose to improved outcomes.

> *"George, we've completed your examination. You've had all your x-rays, and your lab tests are in, and my diagnosis is that you have appendicitis. Now, no one is perfect. I'm a human being, you're a human being.* [I'm working on rapport all the time. I'm going to use everything I know as a hypnotist to stay in rapport with my patient, because I want these words to gain power. Now, here's our commonality:] *"Nobody is perfect. Some things we know to be true.* [Now I stand in the certainty place] *Some things are true and that's just the way it is. And that's certain. But other things are less certain.* [Now I stand in the uncertainty place] *Medicine is not an exact science."*

So, what have I done here? I just proved that certainty is not here in this place [step toward the patient]. Uncertainty is here [step to the side]. I'm going to set up patterns, and I'm going to stack certain things here in *this* place (gesturing), and I'm going to stack other things there in *that* place (gesturing). I would do it this way frequently in the ER and say, *"On the one hand* [Certainty], *there are things we know to be true, and about which we can have absolute certainty and, on the other hand* [Uncertainty], *there are things we are unsure about, that we don't know, that we can only make educated guesses about* (gesturing side to side)." Or, I could say something like this under another circumstance: *"There are some things that happen to some people, and other things that happen to other people."* It is such a simple technique to use, such an easy way that I used to think, "Gosh, there must be a better, more tricky way." You really don't need a more tricky way. You have two hands: on the one hand," and "on the other hand" [gesturing]. What are you doing? You're setting up visual signs for knowledge and truth [one hand], uncertainty and doubt [other hand]. It is going to affect *you* [one hand], going to affect *others* [the other hand]. That is where the artistry of information delivery comes in, which is Part 3 of your patient-doctor encounter.

If you are using the general referential index to say things happen to "other people" without directly suggesting that it will happen to *them*, it works out fine. Let *them* attach meaning. Remember, I told you that when I'm addressing a kid to get ready for an operation, I'm never talking *about* the kid. I'll say, "You know I had a patient *here*" (and I'll always change gender). *"I had a little boy, he was actually a bit younger"* (so that *this* little girl is old). The kid will attach meaning to it. In this context, I want to make sure I don't use the word "you" to direct a negative at that person, because they will hear it that way. You students are sensitive enough now to know when you say "you" to a patient, "That means *you*," they will take it to heart. You want to be careful to avoid saying that. Rather, say, *"I'm a human and you're a human; there are some things we know, and there are some things we don't know. My diagnosis of your condition, at this point in time, is acute appendicitis. What we* know *is this:* (and I'm going to stack this over "here"; [gesturing to the "certain" side]) *You have a fever and a white count of 10,000, and the ultrasound strongly suggests you have an inflammatory mass, and this could be an appendix, or this could be certain other things. What we do know is that when there is the real risk of appendicitis, certain people* [now gesture to the side], *rarely but sometimes, rupture. A rupture could cause infection, and some people, although rare, I'll tell you truthfully that I have never seen it – even die. Those are the risks, but on the other hand* [now gesture toward the patient], *we know that in cases where there is appendicitis, and a good surgery is done,* you *have a good outcome."* That is an embedded suggestion that *you* will have a good outcome.

Eye contact is used a lot for emphasis, i.e., for analogue marking. You don't need to look them in the eye, unless you want to emphasize something. It's not necessary to look them in the eyes all the way through. You can use everything you've got.

> *"But, what we know is that when you have a good surgery, and good outcome, that all those risks are avoided, and that you'll do well and generally get home within a day or two, and heal very rapidly and quickly. Now, I'm obligated to offer you informed consent, and it's your decision whether or*

not to hear it." He could say "no," and then I'd want to clarify that by asking, "*Are you sure?*" Or, he could say "yes," in which case I would respond, saying, "*As you know* [standing now in the "uncertainty" place], *some people have untoward consequences of surgery, but it is very, very rare, and with the surgeon I'm recommending today, I have never seen these consequences*" (if that's true). "*He has the best surgical record, but all surgery can be associated with bleeding, and can carry the risk of bleeding or infection, or even accidents of anesthesia, but they are very, very rare.*

"*On the other hand* [standing now in the "certainty" place], *I have a lot of patients, diagnosed right here, very much like yourself, who have submitted to this procedure, and have had perfect surgery, and have been up and around in no time. The risk of not doing the surgery is rupture. The benefit of doing the surgery is that you will get well. You won't ever have to worry about having appendicitis. Your appendicitis worries are over for life. It's a vaccination against appendicitis, and the benefits are that all the untoward consequences of not treating this disappear. And, in my professional judgment, your condition is such that it warrants surgery, and it warrants surgery now.*" I usually end with, "*I'm here and I'm staying with you. You may not see me, but I'm in this office, here at your beck and call. If you need me, just call me and I'll be there. And, I'm sure, with Doctor Bartan doing the surgery, you'll have a good outcome. Do you have any questions?*"

It's a very simple thing, but it's going to matter more for your patients than anything else you do. You can count on that. Giving informed consent is all about giving the negatives, putting the risks out *here* [gesturing], putting the benefits over *here* [gesturing], staying honest. I was shocked when I saw on the cover of *Time* magazine, "One out of ten American women will have breast cancer." I thought to myself, "That's a great way to create hysteria in the United States." But what about *this* cover: "Nine out of ten American women will not have breast cancer." It's the same thing. So the next part of learning to give informed consent is to understand the nature of statistical information.

Statistical information is *never* about an individual; that's the most important thing to know. Statistical information is always about *groups*. So, nobody, no one person, ever has a 40% chance of survival. That is a common misunderstanding of what statistical information is. A *group* has a 40% chance of survival, 40 out of 100, in a *group*. The reason this is important is because all of the studies you're going to read about are going to color your understanding of these various things. Let's say that 1% of all appendicitis turns out to be a Meckles' diverticulum. That doesn't mean *your patient* has a 1% chance. You don't know what the entry criteria were in the study that established that statistic. Or, even if you do, *he* is not a part of it because *he* didn't have a doctor like you doing an informed consent like you do, and that distinguishes *him*. Maybe the study group was all women; maybe the group was all men. Maybe it was all veterans over the age of 40. As an example, in women's medicine, a lot of the information we have on cardiac illness, and on the treatment of cardiovascular diseases, especially hypertension, is derived from male populations in VA hospitals. So, you can't go to *any* woman and say, "*You* have a 13% chance of stroke." *She* wasn't in that group. *She* doesn't meet the entry criteria. Patients will say, "What are my chances?" and I always tell them, *"I don't know, and no one really knows, but what I do know is that your chances are going to be determined in part by how well we manage this situation, and you're not alone; I'm here with you, and I will stay with you all the way to wellness."*

Let's say there is a 90% death rate from a procedure. What are you going to tell this guy? You're going to say, *"Ten percent of people survive."* He understands what that means, everybody understands what that means, but *how* you present statistical information is really important. A good friend of mine, is a gynecologist at St. Francis hospital in Illinois. He told me about a woman with terrible cancer sweeping through her pelvis. I asked what he told her and he said, "Oh, I hated to do it, it was a miserable day. I was upset myself, and I told her that she had a 94% chance of dying. I basically told her to get things together and get them in order." He's a really nice guy; it's like he is doing an honest thing, but he screwed up. He should have said, *"The statistical information is that in a specific group of women who were studied. Although it's true they were the same as you in that they were women, they differed in a variety of ways, some of which we might not know. One of them is that I'm your doctor and I'm going to help you, and we're going to start hypnotic treatment as an additive to everything else. You're not in that study group; but, even in that group, six out of 100 of them, even without hypnosis, survive."*

Do you hear what I just said? I did not say *"survived,"* because I can change the tense, or make a syntactical error, in order to embed a suggestion. Every time you do that, it's picked up unconsciously. Whenever you break a pattern, whenever there's a non-sequitur or syntactical violation of any kind, it goes right into their unconscious.

Remember that my thesis is that you're doing hypnosis all the time. I know that because I know that a doctor with a white smock on, who doesn't know anything about hypnosis, who gives a sugar pill, and doesn't even know it's a sugar pill, can make 30% of the people in a clinical study get well. In clinical studies, these guys aren't quacks, they're honest, good guys. They've just been handed a placebo: it's double-blinded, and in a double-blinded study, both the doctor and the patient are unaware of who gets what agent.

Let's recap on informed consent. Offer the waiver. That's step one. Set up *certainty* and *uncertainty*, *you* and *them*. It's easiest to do this by *"one hand – and on the other hand."* Remember to begin to embed, mainly by using eye contact, and occasionally point. You can change your voice and make it more of a mandate, stronger, and begin to embed suggestions. This is an advanced course and I'm talking about embedded suggestions. You can feel it when I'm embedding it. It feels different when you get such a suggestion. If I need someone to really pay attention, doesn't she know I'm saying, "pay attention" when I make eye contact with her? It is because it all falls together. Remember that hypnosis is a refinement of every day communications; these are just refinements.

In cases where informed consent is not waived, proceed as follows. Assume for example, you have diagnosed the patient, John, as having an acute abdomen/rule-out appendicitis, and you are recommending surgery. *"Well, John, your tests are in and I would like to tell you my diagnosis and proposed treatment plan. You have already told me you want to know all the pros and cons of any treatment, so that is what I will do. Then you can make an informed decision about your health. Is that alright?"* He says "yes," and you continue. *"First, please understand that there are some things about which we in medicine are* [step forward onto the "certainty" space] *absolutely certain and without doubt. For example,* [stay on the "certainty" space] *your name is John, you have abdominal distress, we are doing everything in our powers to help you, and we will.* [Now, step back to the neutral space where you started] *On the other hand,* [now, step one small step laterally onto the "uncertainty" space] *there is much in medicine that is uncertain or unknown. What are the first causes of illness? When is someone completely cured?* [Step back to the neutral zone]. *You have a very tender abdomen and all of your studies are consistent with the diagnosis of appendicitis; which means that I am recommending emergency surgery. On the one hand* [now extend your left palm toward John so that it lies over the certainty space], *you should know, John, that surgery can explore an acute abdomen like yours, successfully remove an inflamed appendix, and restore health rapidly.* [Step forward into certainty] *This is a wonderful part of modern medicine and one I am recommending for you.* (Step back to neutral) *On the other hand,* [now extend your right hand toward "uncertainty"] *some people sometimes experience the rare complications of surgery: which can be bleeding, infection, accidental injury to the bowel or organs, even the rare accidents of anesthesia… which occasionally include even* [step into uncertainty] *sometimes death.* [Step back to neutral] *Now, you will have a very skilled surgeon and I have truly* [step to certainty] *never seen any of these complications in his competent hands. In fact, I have seen many patients just like yourself* [extend left palm toward patient] *undergo successful surgeries, have brilliant outcomes, and be back to work in no time.* [Step to neutral] *But the decision is yours, John. I only need to tell you that time is of the essence and that if we do not do surgery on suspected appendicitis, some patients can go on to rupture their appendix – and that can be a horrible outcome. So,* [step into certainty] *you decide, John, it's your health."*

Now, let's talk about prognosticating. "Okay, so what is going to happen to me, Doc? What's going to happen?" You know how to deliver the statistical part; be sure to frame it right. Frame the positive edge of the statistic. The statistic is: 60% die, 40% survive. Tell her that 40% survive. Does anyone have an ethical problem with that? People say to me in classes, "Yeah, but aren't you lying to them?" No. I think the gynecologist was lying when he said that 94% are going to die. It would be better to say, *"Six percent of the people, very much like you, get through this. Only you have more than they do, you aren't even in their group. You have me, you have hypnosis, you have a loving family, you have advanced techniques, and that study was three years ago. You have a lot more. I will get through this with you."* Here is what every patient wants to know: "Has anyone ever made it out?" "Has anyone ever got through this thing? I don't care if it is 1 or 100, if someone has made it, I'm making it."

They also want to know that you think they will make it. Moreover, they're going to want to know if you have ever seen anyone make it. There is not a condition I am aware of that someone hasn't survived. This will surprise you, but there are people with juvenile onset, insulin-dependent diabetes who outgrow it. You will not hear that in this medical school, but it's true.

Now, if I'm working with someone, and I know they are going to go outside and hear a spattering of negatives, I'm going to want my "linkage" to cover those negatives, so that I don't lose power. Her mother is going to say this, her best friend is going to say that, the other doctor is going to say the other, and the better I am at future pacing (pacing what their future contains), the more power I retain over those future events. It is critical, because you are not alone in this world, and other people *will* misspeak. What you need to say is, *"Now, you may hear a host of things out there, from a lot of well-meaning people, and many who seem like authorities, and they may tell you that you are going to die, or that you are going to have pain, or you're going to have an unfavorable outcome. What I want you to understand is that they are doing their best, and that the other patients they were wrong about didn't go back to them. They haven't had the benefit of seeing a larger picture, so they have a skewed view of who lives, and who doesn't. And, while that doctor is very well-known in the field, where that friend of yours has been right so many times, or where your mother was so frequently and often wrong in your childhood, I'm telling you something that I now know is certain: "You can survive this. You can get through this."*

So, there you have it. The principles are simple and wholly logical. Your patient's welfare is at stake and your self-image as a doctor will be enhanced. You have nothing to lose and your patients have much to gain by your use of these principles.

Author's note:

> To the extent that patients perceive the clinician as an authority figure, both overt and covert communications may have a marked influence on the patient's experience. This factor,

coupled with the possibility of misunderstanding or misinter-pretation, puts the patient at risk and the concepts presented above go a long way toward minimizing that risk.

Part III

Specific Procedures

Chapter Ten

Principles of Trance Induction

Although most, if not all, hypnotic phenomena can be elicited without requiring a formal trance induction, the trance state is unique in multiple ways and has characteristics that justify taking the time to guide the patient into the state. Induction procedures commonly require several minutes, with some, such as those engaged by Esdale (1850), who employed uneducated workers to perform "passes" over the patient's body, sometimes for hours. To be sure, deepening the state may require a few moments following the initial induction phase, yet the induction itself, in the clinical setting, can be accomplished in just moments. Each clinician will develop techniques that are unique to him or her, and that is as it should be, because they will be more effective when using the technique that is most comfortable. Nevertheless, the principles in the following paragraphs prevail.

It is generally conceded that hypnotic phenomena, possibly including trance, are spontaneously experienced a great many times in life without being identified as hypnosis. We all know the experience of going to a movie and having the rest of the world disappear for a couple of hours, or perhaps we remember how our mind kept "wandering off" when we were at school and trying to listen to the teacher. In the clinical setting, trance is elicited on a premeditated, deliberate basis, usually for a specific purpose.

The available selection of techniques of trance induction is endless, with the most effective being that technique the therapist *expects* to be the most effective. Delivery is far more important than content. The clinician who expects the patient to respond to a brief induction will be just as effective as one who expects that a longer procedure will be more effective. Expectation, experienced by the clinician, is communicated to the patient in multiple ways: by words, gesture, intonation, and emphasis, as well as by many non-verbal communications. To the extent positive expectation is communicated, it is effective in eliciting the desired response.

The word "expectation" has come to have special meaning for me. It seems that what we expect in life is generally what we experience. If the patient expects to experience whatever is suggested, it is apt to be experienced. If the therapist expects to be successful in guiding the patient, success is likely. Thus, it becomes the task of the therapist, fortified by his or her own expectations, to guide the patient to expect the clinical outcome. Expectation comes largely from experience, with training being the place to start. We "expect" to be able to walk across the room, and that expectation came from experience that was not available before we knew how to walk. In like manner, the skill of guiding a patient into trance begins with the clinician learning technique, and then practice generates expectation, with consequent smooth delivery and effectiveness.

We know trance inductions need not be verbal, although clinically that will probably be the most common approach. Nevertheless, it seems important to acknowledge nonverbal induction in understanding the multiple phenomena of hypnosis. James Esdale (1850), a British surgeon working in India early in the 1840s, employed "passes" over the body as hypnotic induction to accomplish anesthesia in over 1,000 successive, surgical procedures – and then published his work. These passes consisted of slow, non-touching motions of the hands of the "hypnotist" over the supine body of the patient, from the head to the feet, accomplished by assistants for periods of many minutes-to-hours preceding surgery. Perhaps the extreme of nonverbal inductions is a technique employed by a few entertainers early in the twentieth century. The "hypnotist" would apply bilateral pressure to the carotid arteries of a standing subject and command "sleep" when the subject began to collapse. One might say resistance was effectively bypassed with this technique. Even in current clinical situations, nonverbal communication in the form of gentle gestures, such as indicating that eyes should be closed, can be effective in altering the patient's mental state.

We also know induction can be covert, as well as overt. The simplest of all inductions is to ask subjects to close their eyes. Just closing their eyes induces an altered state of awareness because the rich flow of information normally present visually has been interrupted, forcing attention on other perceptions. If attention is then called to those other perceptions (perceptions that *must* be present), the subject is guided to take a second step. If attention is then suggested/directed onto another, perhaps unexpected experience such as a memory, the subject is guided further into an altered state and is also becoming increasingly suggestible, the very essence of hypnosis. Of course, suggestibility is present under other conditions, as previously described, and such conditions can also be utilized as the beginning of covert inductions.

Three discrete elements seem to be common to all inductions:

1. There must be some form of communication.
2. There must be a focus of attention on the part of the subject.
3. There must be suggestion for experience, either implied or specified.

Some Observable Signs of Trance

As expanded upon in Chapter 3, changes in the physical attributes of the patient become apparent as he or she enters trance. These observable "signs" can be of value to the clinician in determining the status of the patient and are listed below for reference.

- Absence of skeletal muscle tension
- Absence of volitional movement
- Absence of the swallow reflex
- Eye roll
- Diaphragmatic breathing
- Soft-spoken responses

Not all of these signs need be present; it is a pattern of such signs that indicates trance.

Examples of Induction Procedures

A number of illustrative procedures for trance induction are presented in following paragraphs. They may be employed verbatim or, preferably, modified to fit the clinician's personal way of phrasing things (yet conforming to the language of hypnosis). In all cases, it is advisable to first prepare the patient by identifying and responding to any concerns about the experience of hypnosis, because any fear of the experience will almost certainly interfere with the experience. A therapist can talk about the influence of the entertainer in distorting the reality of hypnosis for purposes of entertainment, and talk about how distortions are commonly communicated through movies and traditional views. It should be stated that hypnosis is truly a way of *gaining* control, not of losing it, responding reassuringly to any concerns expressed by the patient.

The instructions outlined here are simplified and the clinician must use the techniques as indicated for a particular patient, sometimes repeating, and always pacing, the words accordingly, while observing the signs of trance as they develop.

A Four-Step Induction

This procedure is the one I most commonly use in my practice. It seems to be the most effective for the majority of people, it is wholly permissive and, by reviewing the four steps of the procedure with the patient in advance, the clinician can provide reassurance and enhance rapport. It is also the technique I teach my patients as a means of entering trance without assistance, i.e., self-hypnosis. This is a rapid induction technique, a version of which you may find in the literature under "eye closure" technique, and which is an adaptation of the work of Elman (1964).

The patient should be guided through the following four steps, with the therapist pacing the events as compliance is observed, using words similar to these:

1. *Please, when you are ready, close your eyes.*

2. *Now, engage your imagination. Play a game with yourself; imagine/ make believe/pretend those eyes just won't open at all. Maybe, pretend you are a little child again, and part of the game is that you have these eyes that just won't open at all, that are absolutely glued closed.*

3. *And now, while you continue to pretend those eyes won't open, that they are glued closed, I invite you to try to open them, and you will find they just will not open at all. That's it; try hard to open them so*

you know they will not open. (Observe the action of the eye muscles as the opening attempt is made or, if no action is apparent, ask if the patient is trying to open them – seeking an affirmative answer that indicates compliance, and therefore trance.)

4. *Good, now relax your eyes and permit that feeling of relaxation to flow down through your body, all the way down to your toes.*

Note:

If the patient seems at all hesitant to experience hypnosis, or if the therapist senses that the patient is sensitive to the issue of loss of control, the therapist should grant permission, and even encouragement, in advance, for the patient to open his or her eyes during the induction. After initially describing Step 3, in the preliminary introduction, the clinician might say something like this:

As you do this, you will always be fully alert and aware. You will not lose control in any way at all, and if you need to prove to yourself that you are in control, I want you to do that. I want you to stop pretending and open your eyes to show yourself you are in control. Then, knowing you are in control, I will guide you back to Step 1, because I want you to have the skill I am teaching you.

Eye Fixation

Eye fixation is another method of achieving trance, a method that does not require the use of imagination on the part of the patient. The following is an example of what you might say in order to utilize it:

Make yourself comfortable there in your chair. Roll your eyes upward, just as far upward as you can roll them. Now, select some point there on the ceiling and focus your attention on that point. Select some point that is near the upper limit of your range of vision.... As you continue to focus your attention on that point, your eyes will begin to feel stressed and you will want to close them. Please resist that desire, keeping them open and focused on that point, until the need to close them is very strong. Then, when you have decided they are so uncomfortable that you simply must close them, close them in the following way: Close your eyelids slowly downward over your eyes, keeping your eyes rotated upward under the lids, as though they are continuing to focus on that spot on the ceiling. (After observing the eyes close) *"That's fine, now relax your eyes completely and allow your entire body to relax with them.*

Progressive Relaxation

This technique is useful if previous techniques have failed. The technique leaves the entire burden of responsibility with the patient and is purely physical as subjectively experienced by the patient. I like to say:

Make yourself comfortable and take a few deep breaths... and as you breathe in and breathe out, notice that you are becoming more relaxed, that with every breath you release, you release a little more tension... and you can close your eyes so that you can become more aware of your body... and as you do this you notice your body is becoming more relaxed.... Concentrate on your toes and feet... you may feel some tingling, as they relax completely... and let the tension flow out of your body... and the relaxation spreads through the ankles, and calves, and the muscles there relax.... Now, think of your knees and thighs... and, as they relax, you find your thoughts drifting and you are finding an inner peace.... And, the relaxation spreads to the hips... and when the hips feel completely relaxed, I want you to gently nod your head up and down to let me know.... Good... and the relaxation spreads to the pelvis and abdomen.... Let your abdomen relax completely, and your back.... And the soothing deep comfort spreads into the chest... and again you notice your breathing, and the tension is going away... in the neck and across the shoulders, the relaxation is reaching the deep muscles... and spreading down the arms to the hands and fingers ... and now your face relaxes.... The muscles around the mouth... the muscles of the jaws, and cheeks, and around the eyes, can relax completely... and, as you take another deep breath, and let it all the way out, and all those tensions go out with it, and you are relaxed from head to toe, inside and outside, and you can enjoy that pleasant, comfortable, relaxing feeling....

Forehead Touch

This technique is of value in situations where the patient is distracted by pain or other stimuli.

Please, close your eyes. In just a moment, I'm going to touch the center of your forehead with my finger tip." (Touch the patient's forehead with the fingernail of one finger, with that finger flexed to avoid undue pressure. Allow the touch to persist as each suggestion is made.) *Notice the sensation there in your forehead, as I keep my finger positioned there. Notice the pressure of my touch. Notice the slight motion, because I can't hold it perfectly still. Notice how the pressure varies slightly, just as the position varies slightly. Notice how the muscles in your body relax as you continue to focus your attention on that location on your forehead, continuing to be aware of the slight variations in pressure, and the slight variations in the position of my finger. And now, notice that you are becoming more and more at peace with yourself and with your world, and that your mind becomes distracted away from yourself, and notice how comfortable you become with every little motion of my fingertip there on your forehead.*

Arm Drop

When I use this technique, I slowly speak the following words:

Sit comfortably in the chair and hold your arm in front of you with the hand held vertically and slightly above your eyes so you are looking at the back of the hand. Stare at one of the fingers, or the thumb.... Fix your gaze on that one finger and, as you do this, you notice the other fingers tend to fade out of focus. As you continue to fix your gaze on that one finger, you'll notice the whole arm is beginning to get heavier... and the longer you stare at that finger, the heavier the arm becomes, finally beginning to drift downward... and, as the arm drifts downward, you will start to go into a deep state of relaxation.... As you follow with your eyes, and as you keep watching that point on your finger, you will begin to notice your eyes are becoming tired and your eyelids becoming heavy.... You may notice blinking, which is natural... and as your arm feels heavier and heavier, and it gradually drifts down and down, towards your lap... you feel more relaxed and calm and tranquil... and when your hand reaches your lap, your eyes can close.... And, when your eyes close, this is a signal for you to relax even more deeply....

Arm Levitation

Although arm levitation is commonly thought of as a trance response, it can be used as a trance induction:

> *Please lean back in your chair and place your hands on your thighs (or the arms of the chair) and concentrate your attention on your hands as you relax your body…. Good, now take a few deep breaths to release any surface tension… and, as you focus your attention on your dominant hand, you may be able to feel the pressure supporting your fingers and hand, and even the texture of the material supporting your fingers and hand… and, as you continue to focus your attention on your hand, you may become aware of other sensations, perhaps a gentle sensation of warmth, or of coolness, or of a gentle tingling sensation, or of any other sensation…. And, as you continue to focus your attention there on your hand, you can even become aware of your pulse, there in your hand… the sensation of the rush of blood into your hand with each beat of your heart, as it thrusts a surge of blood into your hand…. Do you feel that gentle pulsing, there in your hand?* (It is important to obtain an affirmative response at this point. Repeat the suggestions in different words until you obtain it.) *Good. And now, as you continue to keep your attention focused on your hand, you may also notice a pleasant feeling of lightness forming there in your hand, and in your arm. A natural feeling, a pleasant feeling, a feeling of lightness that increases as the moments go by… and increases with every breath you take… and as the feeling of lightness increases, it can increase to the point that the hand and arm feel so light it is as if they want to begin to rise up in the air…. Do you feel that feeling?* (Again, it is important that you obtain an affirmative response.) *Good. And, as the feeling of lightness increases, your hand feels so light that it will actually begin to rise up into the air…. That's it, higher and higher…. It's as though it rises higher and higher with each breath you take…. Rising higher and higher… and as the hand rises higher and higher, you will find that you slip deeper and deeper into trance… pleasantly and naturally… deeper and deeper into trance…. And now, as your hand begins to drift lower and lower, back to its place of rest, you can slip even deeper into that pleasant, relaxed state we call trance.*

Coin Drop

A coin is placed in the palm of the subject's hand with the arm outstretched in front, as the therapist says:

Concentrate on the coin in your hand and take a few deep breaths, and deliberately relax your body.... As you watch the coin closely, you will notice your hand begin to rotate ... all by itself ... without your doing anything to cause it to happen. And it continues to rotate ... as you become more relaxed ... continue relaxing and breathing and concentrating on the coin as the hand turns more and more.... And, when you are completely relaxed, the coin will drop onto the floor ... and your eyelids will feel heavy and you will close your eyes and become deeply relaxed.... When the coin drops to the floor, you may forget about the coin ... and your hand will descend onto your lap, and you will be in a deep, comfortable and relaxed state....

An alternate strategy is for the patient to hold the coin between thumb and forefinger, and to suggest that the coin gets heavier and heavier and *"... when you are ready, the coin will drop, which will signal the beginning of a deep trance."*

Imagery

Imagery is a favorite of many clinicians. You might say:

Think about a favorite place ... somewhere you would like to be. It might be easier to close your eyes, or you can leave them open ... until you close them, or they close by themselves.... (It often helps to talk about the special place before induction, although the place may change as the induction proceeds.) *Now, you can take some deep breaths, slowly letting them out, and with each breath allow yourself to feel more relaxed ... And now feel yourself in that favorite place ... Imagine that you are there.... Are you there, in that favorite place?* (The subject will usually nod, or perhaps use finger movement to indicate yes. If there is no acknowledgement of your question, repeat the question until there is a response.) *Look around and be aware of what is there – of color, and of light, and of beauty. Perhaps you feel like floating.... Listen to any sounds.... Perhaps you may hear your favorite music.... If you are in the sun, feel the warmth of the sun on your skin.... Smell the fresh air.... You feel so comfortable and safe ... and as you look around your favorite place, and as you become more and more relaxed, you can allow your mind to be at peace....*

Self-controlled

This technique is particularly useful when the patient seems inclined to consciously defy the process, yet the therapist considers it important for trance to be experienced. I might say:

Place your hands there on your thighs, palms down, and allow them to remain quiet for a few moments.... Now, take a deep breath, let it out slowly, and close your eyes.... In a moment – not yet, but in a moment – I'm going to ask that you keep your eyes closed as you begin to slowly lift your right hand (or left, if dominant) and to begin to rotate that hand in such a way that the fingers are pointing toward your forehead. I want to emphasize that you must do this very slowly, and I will verbally guide you to do so.

Now, if you will, please begin to lift that hand, very, very slowly.... That's it. (It is essential that slowness be reinforced, that any acceleration of movement be corrected, so the entire procedure will require at least two-to-three minutes to accomplish.) *I want you to continue to slowly lift that hand, and to slowly rotate that hand, so the fingers point toward your forehead.... And, as your hand slowly lifts, and rotates, and rises toward your forehead, I want you to keep your attention focused on that hand, being aware of just where that hand is out there in front of you... and, as you continue to focus your attention on your hand, being aware of just where it is there in front of you, as it approaches your forehead, I want you to judge, to estimate, just when the tips of your fingers will first touch your forehead.... Estimate the moment of contact, the instant when your fingertips will touch your forehead, and you may find it is as though your fingers and hand pass through your forehead, on into your mind.... And the instant they touch your forehead, I'd like you to be aware of an almost electric sensation that causes your body to release tension, to become instantly and pleasantly relaxed.*

The patient will seldom be able to correctly judge the moment of contact between finger and forehead, and there is a subjective sensation of the finger passing through the forehead. This sensation is reinforced by your suggestions. This focus of attention on the sensation, coupled with the suggestion (implied or otherwise) for trance, will result in the patient slipping into trance.

Chapter Eleven

Hypnosis Attached to Sleep (HATS)

In sleep, which is infinitely more than a mere submergence of waking facilities,
the senses and brain are torpid; the immaterial part of man is vigilant and active.
John D. Quackenbos, M.D. from *Hypnotic Therapeutics*

Introducing Dave Elman

In 1908 John D. Quackenbos, M.D., published *Hypnotic Therapeutics in Theory and Practice*. In this book he spoke at length about "Sleep as a Suggestive State." This contribution, and the contribution of Dave Elman (1964) are the only two published references to the phenomenon that my literature search uncovered. Quackenbos was a physician who was one of the "guiding lights" of hypnosis; he practiced, wrote and lectured extensively on the subject. Elman was a layman who taught the clinical use of hypnosis to clinicians for some 20 years, following a career in entertainment hypnosis. Elman refined and formalized the concept of attaching hypnosis to sleep, making it a practical technique to use. It is a technique I refused to teach for many years, because I considered it to be the technique most subject to misuse by an unprincipled person. Although I still consider it so, I have concluded it is too important not to teach. The fact that an unsuspecting person can be approached, guided into trance without awareness, and influenced by suggestions made while still physiologically asleep, is not to be taken lightly. The reader of this chapter, clinician or otherwise, is implored to use responsible judgment in using, teaching, or even talking about this subject.

Even as a child, I was fascinated by the response of a sleeping play-mate who, when my friends and I gave a command to do something, often obeyed, even though he was asleep. There were many failures, but the successes were sometimes spectacular. Our victim might shout a word, jump up and say something, only to fall fast asleep again, urinate, or cry. We had no understanding of what was happening, only that we could get him to do it, and it was not until my exposure to the teachings of Quackenbos and Elman that I began to understand.

Elman (1964) taught a specific procedure whereby hypnosis could be reliably induced in a sleeping subject. It is basically the protocol I employ today when I elect to attach hypnosis to sleep for some clinical purpose. Although I seldom employ the technique, it does have specific value. Elman's technique is detailed in following paragraphs, which include observations and contributions of my own.

It seems that there are certain levels of sleep in which we are responsive to suggestions. To my knowledge, no research has been done to define those levels, yet it appears that the susceptible level is typically experienced shortly following the transition into sleep. Elman's protocol involves first employing the trance state to achieve natural sleep by means of suggestion, followed by testing the fact of natural sleep by observing physiological changes. When satisfied that natural sleep is being experienced, the clinician attaches hypnosis by means of vocalized suggestions, testing initial responses while doing so. Finally, more meaningful directions are given to the subject as responses are observed and, assuming compliance, therapeutic suggestions are then offered. These suggestions are presented in a more forceful form than the suggestions previously offered as examples in this book.

Encouraging Natural Sleep

Elman taught that it is not possible to translate directly from trance into sleep, that it is necessary to first rouse from trance, then slip into sleep in response to a post-hypnotic suggestion. I have found that to be true on at least some occasions, and so recommend the following sequence. After guiding the supine patient into trance, followed by several compounding exercises to ensure depth, a direct, post-hypnotic suggestion is offered that the patient will sleep in response to a stated cue. A typical suggestion would be:

In a moment, as I count to five, you will find that you rouse from trance. You will rouse feeling refreshed and alert and at peace with yourself and your world. You will also find that when you become aware of my tugging at my earlobe you will suddenly feel very sleepy, and will slip into a deep restful sleep, the kind of deep, restful sleep you have at night, and that will happen every time you become aware of my tugging at my earlobe. Any time, and every time, you become aware of my tugging at my earlobe, you will feel very sleepy, and you will slip into a deep, restful and natural sleep, and you will be guided by this suggestion, even though you have no memory of the suggestion.

After rousing the patient, and bringing up some irrelevant subject for a brief discussion, I execute the cue and the patient reliably responds, doing so within a few moments, and sometimes with a puzzled expression as he or she looks at my hand pulling on my earlobe.

Testing for Natural Sleep

Among the physical changes that take place as a person transitions from being awake to being asleep is decreased respiration rate. This is a reliable indicator and one that is easily tracked; the therapist can time the rate of breathing before rousing from trance, and then compare the rate while in trance to the rate observed while asleep.

The average rate of respiration of a resting adult is on the order of 15 to 18 breaths per minute; the rate of respiration of a sleeping adult will be on the order of 12 to 14 breaths per minute. It is a change in rate that you look for, not the absolute number. Of course, if the clinician is preparing a woman for delivery, her resting rate will be much nearer her sleeping rate, due simply to the restricted transport volume. There may be other variables as well.

Attaching Hypnosis and Testing for Response

Speaking in a clear, quiet voice, address the sleeping patient as follows:

I am Doctor _____, and you can hear me, and you will not wake up. You will remain fast asleep, and you can hear me, and I will know that you hear me when this finger that I am about to touch begins to rise. Even though you hear me, you will remain fast asleep, and I will know that you hear me when this finger begins to rise. The clinician should touch an accessible finger, then wait for the response, and repeat the suggestion until a response is obtained.

Offering Clinical Suggestions

After attaching and testing, the therapist phrases suggestions in a manner similar to the following:

You can hear me, and you will remain deeply and naturally asleep. You can hear me, and in a moment I will say the word "now." Just 10 seconds after you hear me say that word, you will wake up, wide awake, feeling rested and alert, and you will be curious to notice that the tip of your left big toe has begun to itch, and the more you try to scratch it, the more it will itch, until you tell me about it. Then the itching will cease. And any time, and every time, you become aware of my tugging at my earlobe, you will immediately fall fast asleep, the kind of sleep you have at night, restful, natural sleep." And that will be true beginning... "now...."

The clinician should speak the last word distinctly.

Rousing the Patient from HATS

In a moment, I will again say the word 'now,' and just 10 seconds after I say that word, you will wake up, wide awake, feeling alert and rested, and you will remember all you choose to remember, just 10 seconds from... "now...."

Clinical Uses

Because of the unusually reliable, literal responses to suggestions delivered in HATS, and the attendant risk of negative consequences from unintended error on the part of the clinician, I limit my use of this technique to surgical and obstetrical preparation, and to rare instances where uncovering is not otherwise forthcoming. Much is unknown about HATS and caution is indicated.

Chapter Twelve

Subliminal Therapy

The unconscious is highly separate from the conscious mind,
With its own awareness, interests, responses and learnings.

Milton H. Erickson, M.D.

The concepts of mental organization and functioning that evolved into Subliminal Therapy were conceived in the early 1970s, with the first copyrighted paper in 1976. Since then, the protocol has been revised many times and I have employed the evolving process in well over a thousand cases, seldom failing to accomplish the goals set by the patients. I know of no other treatment modality that can claim such success. Its development has dominated my professional life since its conception.

I consider Subliminal Therapy to be a hypnotic technique because, although a formal trance induction is not necessary for its use, patients typically slip into trance during treatment. Subliminal Therapy is an easily learned analytical protocol, used to identify the cause of problems, thereby to resolve their symptoms. The technique is unusual in that the clinician interacts directly with the unconscious domain of the patient's mind with the patient's full conscious awareness and cooperation. Yet, it is truly unique in one respect: The assumption of the existence of Centrum, soon to be defined, and the utilization of Centrum to accomplish desired change. The concepts of subdivided mental functioning and the utilization of unconscious abilities in therapy are well established in the literature.

Subliminal Therapy is an intellectually challenging technique for clinicians. It is consistently rewarding to observe the rapid changes that are accomplished, and it is a technique that has been enthusiastically received in all of the trainings I have conducted.

The process of Subliminal Therapy employs unconscious abilities to review memories of life's experiences, extract relevant data, relate cause and effect, creatively evaluate and devise new solutions, and execute decisions to accomplish the therapeutic goal. All of this is accomplished in a logical progression of questions, requests and responses. The therapist interacts in a direct, logical way, guiding the patient to utilize abilities that are not generally known to the patient. Past views of unconscious functioning as automatic, or as a servo-mechanism, memory bank, and regulator of autonomous processes, are inadequate to explain the phenomena elicited by this technique.

The unconscious elements identified and addressed as independent entities in the course of employing this technique are addressed on a first-person basis to facilitate application of the technique. The unusual nature of this procedure, communicating directly with unconscious entities, is generally accommodated without hesitation or question by the patient. However, initial adjustment on the part of the therapist may be required because of the dramatic shift from conventional approaches.

Theory and Assumptions

The superstructure of Subliminal Therapy rests on four assumptions. First, intelligent unconscious capability exists. Second, the unconscious domain can communicate with consciousness in identifiable ways. Third, the unconscious consists largely of subsystems or "parts" which may function autonomously. Fourth, there is, in the unconscious domain, an entity that may best be described as a "higher self," an entity that cannot be well defined, yet is easily authenticated subjectively. This entity, which I have named "Centrum," functions with some authority within the unconscious domain, communicating with the different parts, and serving as a source of influence on the processes taking place there.

The first assumption – that of unconscious intelligence – has been recognized by Erickson (1989b), among many others:

> *"It is very important for a person to know their unconscious is smarter than they are. There is greater wealth of stored material in the unconscious. We know the unconscious can do things, and it's important to assure your patient that it can. They have to be willing to let their*

unconscious do things and not depend so much on their conscious mind. This is a great aid to their functioning."

In Subliminal Therapy, patients are taught to allow their unconscious minds to work in a logical, organized, sequential process, guided by the therapist, or under some conditions self-guided by the patient.

The second assumption is that Centrum can communicate with the patient at a conscious level of awareness and, through the patient, can communicate with the therapist. This inner-patient communication from Centrum to conscious awareness may be facilitated by means of ideomotor signals, as classically described by Cheek (1994), via other ideosensory means such as an imagined chalkboard on which Centrum is requested to write, by an inner voice, or by subjectively perceived physical sensations as taught by Bandler and Grinder (1979). The viability of ideomotor signals has been well documented by Erickson (1989b) as well as by Cheek and LeCron (1968), who have described the use of finger signals and Chevreul's pendulum for that purpose. The phenomena of memory itself can be considered an illustration of unconscious-to-conscious communication, in that memories are consciously perceived via the senses.

The third assumption is that the unconscious mind is made up of multiple "parts." The literature is rich with examples of recognition of the existence of such parts. Hilgard (1978) states, "Personality is much less unified than we would like to believe and volition is subject to dissociation just as are perceptual processes." James' (1890) assertion that "Consciousness is split into parts that ignore each other," and Janet's (1907) interpretation that "systems of ideas are split off from the major personality, unconscious but capable of becoming represented in consciousness through hypnosis," support this concept. Green (1977) described, "...the autonomous entities working for themselves as unconscious parts of our psyche." Subliminal Therapy enlists these "autonomous entities" for therapeutic purpose. In this respect, Subliminal Therapy is also similar to Assagioli's *Psychosynthesis* (1965), which is described as a process of integration of the parts of the psyche, and to Watkins' (1979) *Ego State Therapy*, in which various "states" are "cathected."

The fourth assumption – that of the existence of "Centrum" – is less easily defended by reference to the literature. The existence of a Higher Self, hereafter referred to as Centrum, was originally assumed as an explanation for various phenomena observed clinically, phenomena that defied other explanation. As the services of Centrum are engaged in the process of therapy, communication apparently does take place within the unconscious domain, and continuing practical benefits convincingly validate Centrum's existence. The reader is encouraged to experiment with self and with others to test this assumption by requesting a response from Centrum. For example, you might phrase your request as, *"Centrum, as a way of demonstrating your presence, please respond by creating a distinct sensation some place in my body."*

As engaged in Subliminal Therapy, the capacity for unconscious reasoning, involving intelligent, creative abilities, makes it possible to bypass much of the resistance typically evident in therapy. Moreover, should the therapist so choose, this capacity can free the therapist to conduct the course of therapy without being involved in the content and influences being unconsciously addressed by the patient. In a test of limits, therapy has been successfully conducted without the therapist even knowing the nature of the presenting problem. Even more startling, the patient may not be consciously aware of the mental processes engaged, or of the factors and influences addressed, until such awareness is requested.

In many instances, the technique of Subliminal Therapy can be employed as the sole treatment. However, in some situations, it may be more effectively employed as an adjunct to other modes of treatment. If resistance to therapy is encountered in the use of other interventions, an excursion into the process of Subliminal Therapy may resolve the resistance and permit resumption of the original treatment. In any event, and regardless of the technique being employed in therapy, Subliminal Therapy can be used as a means of systematic uncovering, of measuring progress in therapy, and possibly of testing attainment of the therapeutic goal.

The Procedure

Subliminal Therapy is a step-by-step process in which the therapist guides the patient to use unconscious abilities to investigate the cause of the presenting problem and then to resolve the presenting problem by achieving a mature understanding of the causal influences. Assuming the problem is psychogenic, resolution by this means may reasonably be expected. To enable the therapist to intelligently guide the course of therapy, Centrum is taught to signal the patient when a requested step has been accomplished. This prearranged response is then verbally reported by the patient, or observed if finger signals are employed.

In some cases, the patient may have, either consciously or unconsciously, the knowledge and skills necessary to resolve the problem once the cause is uncovered. If this is the case, the function of the therapist is only to guide the patient through the structured process of the therapy. In other instances, the patient may lack the knowledge and/or the skills required, and so the role of the therapist becomes that of educator, in addition to guide. If education is not required, the therapeutic goal may often be accomplished within minutes after the therapist provides initial orientation and instruction. If frequent intervention and support by the therapist is required, therapy will require proportionately longer periods of time.

The process is most effectively utilized when the patient has a clearly defined, therapeutic goal. Therefore, the first step taken by the therapist is to ensure clear expression of the goal by the patient and, if necessary, to assist the patient in defining the goal in the form of a simple, verbal statement of desire. Multiple goals may be identified and, if so, priorities of treatment must be defined by the patient.

The therapist next explains the process of Subliminal Therapy by presenting a model of the mind in which concepts of unconscious and conscious organization and capabilities are defined. Many years ago, I created a booklet (Yager, 1985) for my patients, which introduces these concepts. I encourage my patients to read the booklet before therapy begins, thereby reducing one-on-one time. In this model of the mind, the unconscious is described as

consisting of multiple "parts," each having a function and purpose, and each having come into existence when that function
was "learned" during the course of experiences over a lifetime. I
explain that humans generally function pretty well, which is evidence that a guiding entity must reside in the unconscious domain,
an entity that communicates with other parts of the mind, thereby
providing continuity and direction, influencing experience. This
entity is introduced as "Centrum." Patients readily accommodate
this model of the mind and accept the assertion that the unconscious entities are both well intended and capable of analytical
reasoning.

Patients also readily accept more unusual statements such as,
*"Anything you can do consciously you can do unconsciously, and you
can probably do it better in the unconscious, because there is access to
more information there,"* (Erickson, 1976, p.122) and, the cause of
the problem is in the unconscious. After all, if it were conscious,
you would already have solved it; therefore, the solution must
ultimately take place with unconscious assistance.

When the patient is familiar with this model of the mind, instruction is provided about how to perceive communications from the
unconscious domain. This perception is required for the therapist
to communicate with Centrum. It is explained that communication
to Centrum takes place "even as you hear me speaking," and that
communication *from* Centrum must come through the patient's
conscious perceptions. Early in the development of Subliminal
Therapy, ideomotor signals and Chevruel's pendulum were used
as the vehicle of this communication. My experience has shown
that it is more practical, flexible, and efficient to request the patient
to form a mental image of a chalkboard, on which Centrum can
write answers to the therapist's questions and requests. The patient
is instructed to simply "observe" the chalkboard and to report *only*
what appears there.

At this point in the process, the patient typically and spontaneously slips into an altered state of awareness that is identifiable
as hypnotic trance. This state is evidenced by eye closure and roll,
flaccid muscle tone, diaphragmatic breathing, and general physical calmness. Such physical demonstration is not always evident;
many patients continue to function with their usual mannerisms,

with only a "dreamlike," unfocused appearance to their eyes, as they perceive the unconscious communications.

The most frequently encountered obstacle in the use of Subliminal Therapy is a tendency on the part of some patients to report cognitive opinions in lieu of communications from Centrum. Common problems are the patient's giving reports biased by a desire to please, or by conscious disagreement with the answers actually perceived. The therapist is urged to spend a fair amount of time emphasizing to the patient that although there may be disagreement with the answers perceived, or impatience with delay in unconscious responses, or a wish to please, time and money will be wasted unless reports include *fully* and *only* what appears on the chalkboard. With minimal practice, the therapist learns to sense cognitive responses by the way the words are presented or emphasized – "I think…" or "Well, …" or "I don't believe so" are obvious examples of cognitive responses. A simple "yes" or "no" or "now" or "yes and no" are apt to be valid responses from Centrum, as are the expressions: "It says…" and "There's a 'yes' and a 'no'."

From patient to patient, some variation in time will be evident between question (or request) and responses from Centrum. Most responses will occur in the order of a few seconds, yet a few might require a minute or more. When the response is slow, patience on the part of the therapist is required. The patient is probably experiencing a distortion of time and so is not bothered by the delay. If the therapist is concerned that nothing is happening, a clarifying question can be interjected such as, *"Centrum, are you working on the requested task?"* If the response is "yes," acknowledge the response and simply wait.

To ensure adequate theoretical understanding by the patient of how dysfunctions and limitations can be learned at both conscious and unconscious levels of awareness, the therapist explains: *"You were not born with the problem you have presented; there was a beginning, a first time, and the memory of that first time is retained in your unconscious mind. Centrum has the ability to examine that memory and to learn from it from the perspective of present knowledge, as opposed to the perspective of limited knowledge of that earlier time."* The process is then described to clarify that the dysfunction or limitation began, not as a "problem," but rather as a "solution" to a set of circumstances that were then in effect. Only from the perspective of the present is the dysfunction recognized as a problem. Treatment is further proposed as a method of resolving conflicts by replacing lessons learned and decisions made "then" with lessons and decisions appropriate "now," modifying conditioned responses in consequence.

The therapist explains this theory of learning to the patient in terms of suggestibility and of conditioned response. Suggestibility is explained as a mental condition in which new inputs (suggestions) are internalized and integrated without being subjected to conscious, critical judgment. Hypnosis is explained as an example of such a mental condition, and other examples of suggestibility are offered. For example, *"The small child is exceedingly suggestible, having as yet only a minimal accumulation of knowledge to use as a basis for critical evaluation."* The therapist explains that we are also very suggestible, even as adults, during intense emotional experiences, and also when we are confused. Such mental conditions allow occasional "learning" of undesired behaviors, as well as the constructive learning that takes place during life.

The phenomenon of conditioning is explained to the patient by referring to Pavlov's experiments with animals, especially those with dogs that were conditioned to respond by salivating to the stimulus of the sound of a bell. The therapist explains that there was, at one time, a rational connection between the stimulus and the response. Food odor was presented coincident with the ringing of a bell and the dog would salivate. This was repeated many times until, even when food was not presented, the dogs would salivate in response to the bell alone. Similarly, an adult who experiences a lifelong fear of the dark, learned such fear in a context in which it was absolutely logical to associate fear with darkness.

The Process

I recommend that the first questions posed to Centrum, for response on the chalkboard or by other ideosensory means, include, *"Centrum are you willing to cooperate as I guide the process toward achievement of your conscious goal?"* and, *"Is that goal advisable, is it supportive of your well-being, is it in your best interests now, in your present situation?"* Assuming an affirmative response, ask if Centrum is willing to do the things necessary to cause the goal to become reality. Although an affirmative response to this question is usually received, there may be an occasional "no." Such negative response usually indicates that some other "part" of the mind is resisting the work, and this resistance must be resolved before progress can be made. Resolution will likely entail identification of the basis for the resistance and education of that "part" regarding current reality. Centrum should be guided to identify, and then to communicate with the resisting part, to thereby resolve the resistance.

The answers to these questions determine the immediate course of therapy. A negative response to either question must be addressed and resolved before further work can be accomplished. Centrum must be persuaded to agree with the conscious goal, or vice versa, and this agreement is best accomplished by the therapist acting as an intermediary between Centrum and consciousness, negotiating such mutual understanding. Encourage the patient to express beliefs and desires and motivations aloud, so that Centrum is able to understand and intelligently rebut. When each fully understands the other, agreement consistently ensues.

Unwillingness to work may stem from Centrum (or some other part) wanting to protect consciousness from unpleasant or traumatic information. This issue is usually handled with a simple question, *"Centrum, are you willing to work without conscious awareness?"* If Centrum is willing to proceed without conscious awareness of the work engaged, I proceed with the patient consciously blind to content. This also, of course, requires the therapist to function with limited feedback; if the patient is blind, so is the therapist. It will probably be possible to achieve conscious awareness of the content after completion of the work, if desired by the patient, or if such awareness is necessary to resolve the problem. Centrum should be asked, *"Does the patient now need awareness to resolve this problem?"*

Assuming Centrum is willing to do the work, the first task requested of Centrum is that of an investigation: Centrum is asked to review, without conscious awareness if necessary, all available memories of experiences and influences that are significant to the patient's present goal and to communicate with all parts that are involved in any way. The purpose of the investigation is explained to be the development, at least at an unconscious level of awareness, of understanding of those influences that are of concern in the present. The therapist requests that this investigation be conducted from the perspective of the knowledge and maturity of the present, so that the understanding obtained is not limited to the perspective of "then." Centrum is requested to indicate when the investigation is complete by causing the word "complete" to be written on the chalkboard.

If the "complete" response is forthcoming, treatment is continued. If no answer is forthcoming, steps necessary to promote that understanding must be taken. Centrum may be led through a step-by-step investigation, beginning with the first sensitizing event and proceeding through succeeding experiences, to achieve understanding of the etiology of the dysfunction. Conscious awareness of related memories may be requested so that informed guidance can be provided by the therapist; however, such awareness may not be forthcoming. Any steps considered appropriate may be taken, limited only by the skill and imagination of the therapist. Fortunately, lack of unconscious understanding of the material addressed is rarely encountered; however, until such understanding is present, it is futile to proceed.

Following the foregoing stage-setting procedures, Centrum is guided through a sequence of steps, leading to the desired change. These steps are detailed in the flowcharts appended to this chapter.

After repeating the sequence of steps in the flowchart to address multiple goals, Centrum will probably be able to proceed with additional goals without the guidance of the therapist. In this event, the therapist poses the question of capability to Centrum by asking, *"Centrum, are you now capable, without further assistance from me, of accomplishing the consciously desired goal?"* If the response is "no," assistance may be provided by the therapist in the form of instructions about communicating with involved parts, and replacing conditioning that were appropriate "then" with conditioning that is appropriate "now." Thus, conditioning is changed; the response can shift from what it had been. Alternatively, Centrum may be requested to employ creative abilities to devise one or more preferred solutions, thereby providing flexibility in resolution. However, since it is essential that Centrum have the necessary abilities if the goal is to be achieved, the creative capacities of the therapist may occasionally be called upon to provide them by instruction and education.

Having been assured of the willingness and ability of Centrum to accomplish the desired goal, the therapist asks that the work be accomplished. This step may seem redundant, the indication for it being implicit in foregoing work; however, it is usually necessary as inaction results without the request. This absence of proactive function is common to every step of this treatment, and those familiar with hypnotic phenomena will recognize it as characteristic of hypnotic response.

Peripheral factors may be significant to the success of the therapy, factors that have not been resolved in the previous steps. The task of the therapist is to ensure that opportunity is provided for Centrum to consider and resolve these concerns. This step is accomplished by asking Centrum if there is more to be done, by taking the necessary steps to complete remaining work, and then repeating the question until the answer is "no."

The key question, *"Centrum, has your goal now been accomplished?"* is then asked. A negative response is indicative that another part of the mind, perhaps without awareness of Centrum, is active in a restrictive way and must be dealt with. Communication between that other part and Centrum may be established simply by request, and may provide resolution of the problem by facilitating mutual understanding between them. Resolution may require that the resisting part be guided to consider the basis of the resistance from the perspective of present reality, thereby affording opportunity to change its position. That the resisting part may not have awareness of present reality may seem incomprehensible; nevertheless, it is possible and even likely. In some cases, unless willing to communicate with Centrum, the part may require guidance through the same therapeutic process as just experienced by Centrum with the therapist interacting directly with the part.

An affirmative response to the preceding question, followed by similar probing questions designed by the therapist, may tentatively satisfy both patient and therapist that the work is indeed complete. As a further test of the completeness of the work, Centrum may be asked to convince the patient of completeness, and/or the patient may be guided to test completeness by imagining a situation in which the desired goal is in effect. Any difficulty in creating this imaginary situation is evidence that the work is not complete, that one or more parts of the mind still resist the desired change. In this case, the therapist repeats the procedure outlined above until the goal appears to be accomplished, and then tests again to affirm accomplishment.

Because the patient is often consciously unaware of the content of the work that has been completed, conscious conviction of completion is seldom expressed. If deemed advisable, conviction may be obtained by requesting Centrum to provide it by causing some experience (an itch, a tickle, a thought, an involuntary movement, etc.), the purpose of which is to convince the patient of completion. The results of this request can be dramatic and occasionally humorous. It is not clear that cognitive conviction is necessary; however, it does seem to have real, if undefined, value when provided.

As the final step, Centrum is requested to provide conscious awareness of the content of the work just accomplished, and of the basis for that work, including memories of related events, understanding, and insight. Such awareness is usually provided and the patient seems to benefit from it. However, the awareness may be denied and the patient may or may not wish to pursue the matter. If desired, pursuit will require employing the same basic procedure as used to address the problem itself to resolve the reason for denial. Some part or parts of the mind are preventing conscious awareness. Those parts must be persuaded to permit it. If the patient is indifferent about knowing, the matter should be dropped and therapy considered provisionally complete.

Note:

The process previously described is only one of many possible protocols. The therapist is not limited to any particular design and is encouraged to tailor the process to the client.

For example, the therapist may conclude that interacting directly with a given "part" may be more appropriate than using Centrum as an intermediary. One part may be enlisted to communicate with another; communication between parts may be accomplished without conscious awareness; or the therapist may or may not insist upon a given request being accomplished. The variations are many.

A Session Transcription

The following is a transcription of a portion of a session with a 25-year-old female. The session was the fourth in a series in which she had addressed several minor issues via Subliminal Therapy and so was familiar with the process. The therapeutic goal addressed was to "eliminate her bulimia."

Responses from Centrum and other unconscious parts, as reported by the patient, are capitalized and immediately follow the questions and requests posed. Comments that have been inserted for clarification are italicized. Remember, although the answers are immediate in the transcript, it is often not true in practice.

Dr.   Centrum, do you support your conscious wish to eliminate the bingeing and purging? YES

> *The reader will note that* Centrum *is addressed in the first person. This practice avoids confusion, expedites the work, and is readily accommodated by the patient.*

Centrum, are you willing to do the necessary work, as I guide the process, toward accomplishing that goal? YES

Then Centrum, please investigate, with or without conscious awareness, all aspects of this goal: Identify the part, or parts, that cause the bingeing and purging and communicate with them to learn of their reasons for doing so. Identify any part that might resist your achievement of your goal. Review memories of related events and do all else necessary for you to understand all possible aspects of this problem. Let me know by writing the word "complete" on the chalkboard when you have completed this task to the limit of your ability. COMPLETE

Centrum, please write on the chalkboard any reason you are bingeing and purging.

GUILT
PEOPLE
SELF-IMAGE
CLEAR GOAL
FEAR

This set of responses was unexpected. Usually only one is forthcoming.

Peggy, do you consciously understand what Centrum means by "guilt?"

Peggy   I think I do…. If I eat inappropriately, I feel guilty. Then I vomit to punish myself.

Dr.   Centrum, is that what you referred to? YES

Peggy, what is your conscious reaction to that? Does it make sense to you?

It is important to obtain conscious opinion and perspective from the patient, rather than for the therapist to provide it.

Peggy   I don't want to feel guilty. I want to eat appropriately, yet I'm confused. When I don't like a part of myself, I punish it.

Although the meaning of this statement is not clear to me, it seems clear to her, so I proceed.

Dr.   Centrum, do you understand why you do that? NO

Centrum, is some part of your mind causing that to happen? YES

Centrum, are you in communication with that part? SOMETIMES

Are you in communication with it now? NO

Are you willing to communicate with that part now? YES

And, Centrum, is that part (or parts, as the case may be) willing to communicate with you? NO

Are those parts willing to receive information, if they can do so without having to respond, without having to expose themselves? CONFUSED

My error. I should have been clearer in my question.

Centrum, I believe that part of your mind is well-intended. I believe it is doing what it is doing for reasons it considers to be in your best interest. I doubt that the part is aware of the consequences of what it is doing. I doubt that it is aware of present reality. I think it is functioning on the basis of what "was," rather than on the basis of what "is." I also believe that part is probably feeling threatened by this work. I want to make it possible for that part to learn about present reality, to catch up with the rest of your mind. If it can do so without threat, by listening only, it may be willing to do so. Therefore, I ask again if the part is willing to receive information for consideration without having to respond? YES

Then Centrum, please communicate to that part your understanding of the present, of the consequences of what it is doing and of the advantages of cooperating with you. Inform that part, educate that part, persuade that part to your way of thinking and let me know by the word "complete" when you have done so. COMPLETE

Centrum, now that the part has received that information, is it willing to communicate fully with you toward mutual understanding? YES

> *Note the continuing emphasis on mutual understanding. It is an underlying theme of this technique.*

Then, Centrum, please communicate further with that part and when there is full mutual understanding, let me know by the word "complete." COMPLETE

Centrum, does that part, or those parts, still want you to punish yourself? NO

Centrum, is it okay for you to know and understand what is going on at a conscious level of awareness? YES

Centrum, please provide that awareness now.

Peggy   It's complete. I was thinking about the other parts being my protection. The others that punished me... They didn't understand.

Dr.   Centrum, do you now have all the conscious understanding you need to eliminate the self-punishment? YES COMMUNICATION

> *The word "communication" was not expected. I assumed it was an indication from Centrum that, although all necessary conscious understanding was there, some kind of communication was still needed.*

Peggy   Centrum says he needs to communicate all information to other parts.

> *My assumption was apparently correct. Also, notice the gender of Centrum is masculine in this case.*

Dr.   Okay, Centrum, please do that. Communicate full understanding to every part of your mind so there can be cooperation. OKAY

Centrum, is there more to be done to eliminate the guilt that is causing the bulimia? LET GO OF GUILT

Again, here is guidance for me from Centrum. To be provided such guidance is the exception, not the rule.

Centrum, do you know how to do that? FORGIVING

And who must be forgiven? OTHER PARTS

Centrum, do you forgive those other parts? YES

And, Peggy, do you consciously forgive them?

Peggy   Yes, I do.

Dr.   Centrum, does any part, for any reason whatsoever, not forgive? NO

Centrum, is there more to be done to eliminate that guilt? NO

Very good. Now, let's address the second of those reasons. Peggy, do you consciously understand what Centrum meant by "people?"

Each of the five stated reasons, guilt, people, self-image, clear goal, and fear, must be addressed in a manner similar to that above. There is bound to be a significant amount of interaction among the five, and it may be necessary to readdress each before the goal is finally achieved.

Research

My experience with hundreds of patients has indicated a high order of efficacy, as have anecdotal reports from others who I have trained in the technique, yet this is only anecdotal evidence. The minimal research that has been accomplished to date is reported in following paragraphs.

Subliminal Therapy was initially tested in 1977 by a review of the clinical records of 41 consecutive patients, of random age and sex, who presented a total of 161 problems, including a wide variety of behavioral, somatic, emotional, phobic, and sexual concerns. I treated these patients on an individual basis, in a private, clinical setting, for an average of 6.2 hours each. Achievement of all therapeutic goals was self-reported a minimum of one-month post-treatment by 13 of the patients (32%), and achievement of at least half of their therapeutic goals by an additional 17 (41%). These results are reported without claim of adequate research controls. The data were compiled, in some cases, months after the therapeutic work was done.

In 1978, a quasi-controlled study was conducted in which three females were treated for hay fever. Following three individual treatment sessions, two reported their symptoms had completely vanished, and the third reported an improvement of 35–40%. The three sessions lasted an average of 21 minutes each, following initial introduction and instruction, so that each subject was seen individually for an average of 63 minutes.

In early 1979, as a test of the theory that the therapist could successfully treat patients without knowing the nature of the presenting problem, five subjects were so treated. With the assistance of a colleague, I was given the first name of the subjects, and information as to whether they wished to eliminate something or achieve something. Only after the conclusion of the study was I made aware of their presenting goals. Four of the five successfully accomplished their goals.

Later in 1979, I conducted a pilot study in which a computerized version of Subliminal Therapy was employed in lieu of a human therapist. Five subjects presenting simple phobias were treated in a context that limited instructions to printed material, contact with the therapist being confined to logistic issues. Four of the five subjects reported successful elimination of their phobias. Two reported success during the first treatment session, one subject required two sessions, and the fourth required three. The duration of treatment sessions, i.e., interaction with the computer, was determined by the subject being treated, and varied from 17 minutes to 48 minutes.

Additionally, Subliminal Therapy has been clinically validated by being employed in the treatment of a wide variety of presenting disorders in hundreds of cases, by multiple therapists.

Flowcharts of the Process of Subliminal Therapy

The following flowcharts are divided into three phases:

- Phase I includes the preliminary steps required to set the stage for the process to follow.

- Phase II includes the four preparatory steps required.

- Phase III is the process itself as presented via a set of flow charts. The first of these charts, the "Basic Flowchart," presents the flow of events from beginning to end of treatment. In the unlikely event the patient should respond in the most expeditious manner, this will be the only chart needed. However, should the patient respond with answers that require deviation into other venues, follow the flow of questions by reference to the charts on succeeding pages.

Note:

Although these charts will be adequate for most patients, there will be responses that do not fit the flow of these charts. In this event, the clinician is challenged to devise a set of logical questions that guide the process until a return to the charts becomes possible.

Following the flowcharts, there is a narrative elaboration of the steps of Subliminal Therapy as detailed in the flowcharts of Phase III. This elaboration includes suggestions that might be employed, as well as explanations of the purpose of each step.

Phase I
Set the Stage

Referring to the introduction booklet (if used), explain the following points to the patient, ensuring understanding of the concepts as you progress.

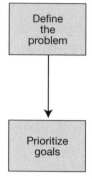

Explain the tasks of the patient at a conscious level (perceiving communications from Centrum on an imaginary chalkboard and communicating those communications to you) and the task of Centrum.

Explain your function as that of a guide and resource as the patient does the work. Ensure that the patient understands his or her conscious responsibility when employing Subliminal Therapy, which is that of reporting to you those communications perceived on the chalkboard, as opposed to communicating conscious opinions. Explain that it will be Centrum's role to communicate with you via the chalkboard and to communicate as necessary with other parts of the mind.

Phase II – step 1
Identify the Goals

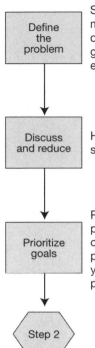

Sometimes a patient presents just one goal, but usually there is more than one. Your task as the therapist is to assist the patient in defining – and often separating – the problems presented. The goals will be the solutions to the problems. If the problem is, for example, "headache," the goal will be "Eliminate the headache."

Having defined the goals, discuss each one to reduce it to a succinct, accurate statement.

Prioritize the sequence of the process according to the patient's priorities unless you have clearly definable reason to suggest otherwise. In the event you do suggest a change, go with the patient's decision after discussion. This will be the order in which you conduct the therapy, accommodating future changes in priorities, additions and deletions as desired by the patient.

(continued)

Phase II – step 2
Education

The patient must be introduced to the theory and concepts of Subliminal Therapy. This can be expedited by use of my booklet for patients, "*Subliminal Therapy: Utilizing the Unconscious Mind,*" but the booklet is not essential. Each of the following concepts must be explained to the satisfaction of the patient and you are cautioned to ensure the patient understands each concept at each step.

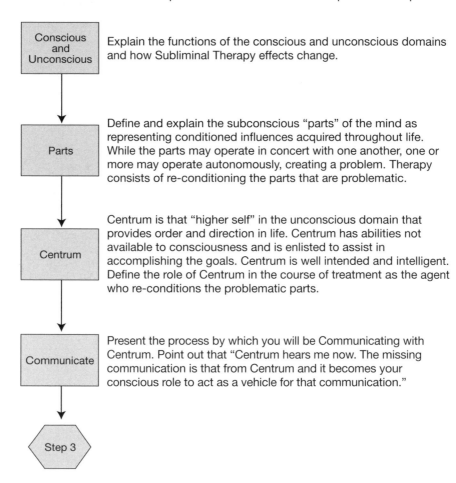

Conscious and Unconscious — Explain the functions of the conscious and unconscious domains and how Subliminal Therapy effects change.

Parts — Define and explain the subconscious "parts" of the mind as representing conditioned influences acquired throughout life. While the parts may operate in concert with one another, one or more may operate autonomously, creating a problem. Therapy consists of re-conditioning the parts that are problematic.

Centrum — Centrum is that "higher self" in the unconscious domain that provides order and direction in life. Centrum has abilities not available to consciousness and is enlisted to assist in accomplishing the goals. Centrum is well intended and intelligent. Define the role of Centrum in the course of treatment as the agent who re-conditions the problematic parts.

Communicate — Present the process by which you will be Communicating with Centrum. Point out that "Centrum hears me now. The missing communication is that from Centrum and it becomes your conscious role to act as a vehicle for that communication."

Step 3

(continued)

Phase II – step 3
Process Instruction

Referring to the introduction booklet (if used), explain the following points to the patient, ensuring understanding of the concepts as you progress.

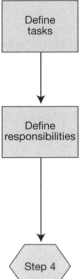

Explain the tasks of the patient at a conscious level (perceiving communications from Centrum on an imaginary chalkboard and communicating those communications to you) and the task of Centrum.

Explain your function as that of a guide and resource as the patient does the work. Ensure that the patient understands his or her conscious responsibility – when employing Subliminal Therapy – is that of reporting to you those communications perceived on the chalkboard, as opposed to communicating conscious opinions. Explain that it will be Centrum's role to communicate with you via the chalkboard and to communicate as necessary with other parts of the mind.

(continued)

Phase II – step 4
Set Up Centrum

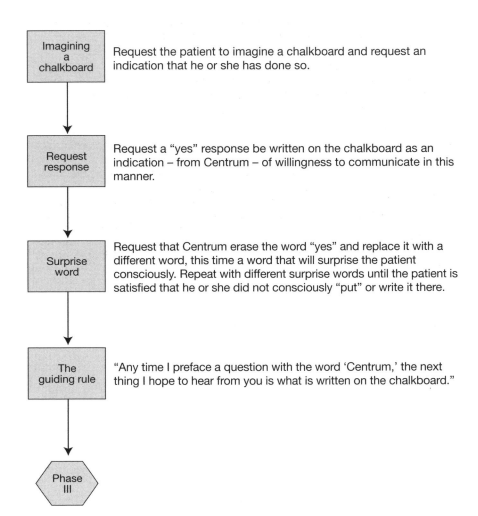

Imagining a chalkboard	Request the patient to imagine a chalkboard and request an indication that he or she has done so.
Request response	Request a "yes" response be written on the chalkboard as an indication – from Centrum – of willingness to communicate in this manner.
Surprise word	Request that Centrum erase the word "yes" and replace it with a different word, this time a word that will surprise the patient consciously. Repeat with different surprise words until the patient is satisfied that he or she did not consciously "put" or write it there.
The guiding rule	"Any time I preface a question with the word 'Centrum,' the next thing I hope to hear from you is what is written on the chalkboard."

Phase III

Phase III
Basic flowchart

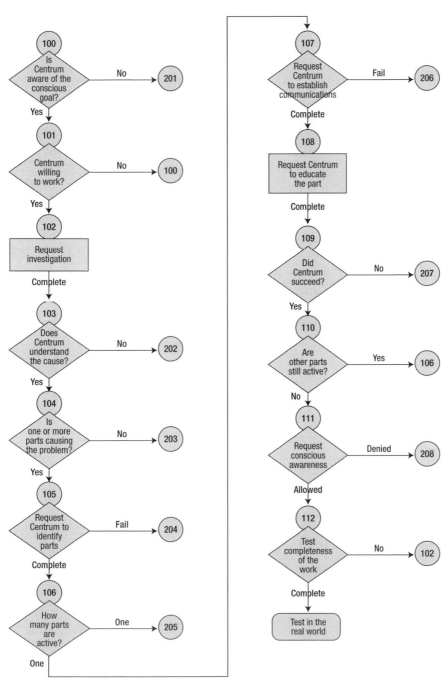

(continued)

Phase III
Excursions

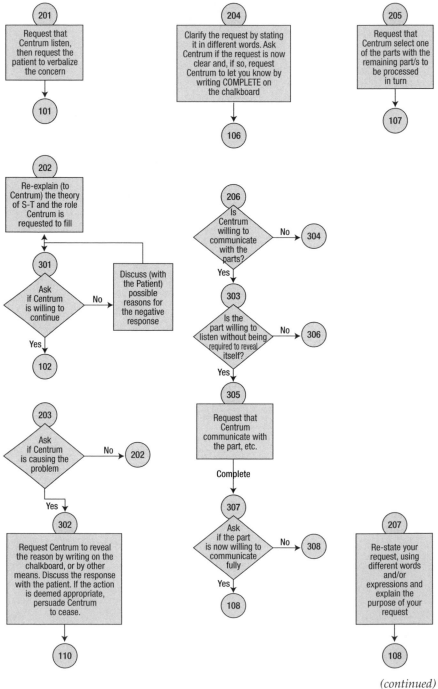

(continued)

Phase III
Excursions

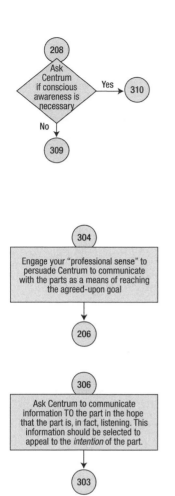

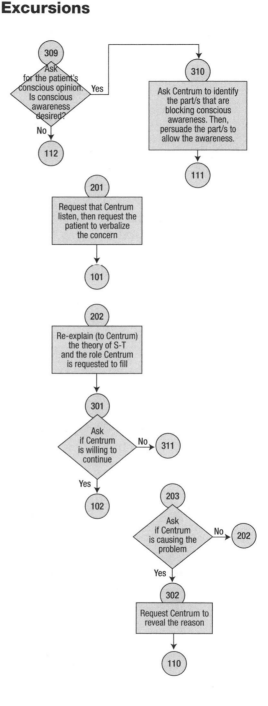

Elaborations

Examples of suggestions are italicized

100 Having set the stage to begin the process of Subliminal Therapy, determine if Centrum is actually aware of the conscious goal to be addressed. Since you are advised to avoid assumptions, insure that Centrum is aware of the conscious goal by asking. Do not assume Centrum is aware. Request that Centrum respond by writing the answer on the chalkboard.

Asking Centrum to indicate completion by writing the work "complete" a few times as you begin the work will make it unnecessary to repeatedly ask for the chalkboard response in the future; the responses will come automatically.

Centrum, are you aware of your conscious desire regarding this (problem)?

101 It is wise to ensure that Centrum is willing to be involved in the process. And if there is a negative response, it will be necessary to persuade Centrum to do so. Here, your talents as a clinician come into play. However, it is rare that Centrum is not cooperative.

Centrum, are you willing to cooperate in this effort, to do some work as I guide you and teach you how to accomplish your conscious goal?

102 Since your intention is to request Centrum to do the work of therapy, first ask Centrum if willing to cooperate and to accomplish the conscious goal. Assuming an affirmative answer, ask Centrum to investigate the roots of the problem and elaborate as necessary to insure that Centrum understands the request. Then ask Centrum if the request is clear. Assuming an affirmative answer, ask Centrum to complete the investigation as comprehensively as possible with the objective of Centrum achieving as complete an understanding as is possible at this time, and to indicate completion of the task by writing the work "complete" on the chalkboard.

Centrum, please investigate this issue. Review memories of events that may have had something to do with it and communicate with those parts that are involved. The objective, Centrum, is for you to understand how this (problem) became part of your life. Centrum, is my request clear to you? (Answer – if yes) Then, Centrum, please complete that task as comprehensively as is possible at this time and let me know when you have done so by writing the word "complete" on the chalkboard

103   Again, no assumptions. Ask Centrum if the investigation produced understanding of the cause of the problem. If not, you must approach the process in a way that will ensure Centrum's understanding.
Centrum, do you now understand the cause of the (problem), how it came to be a part of your life?

104   Ask Centrum if the problem is being caused by one or more parts of the mind. If more than one, you must guide Centrum to interact with each part independently, one at a time, through step 109 of the sequence. Then return to step 107 after completing the education of each part.
Centrum, is the (problem) being caused by the action of one or more parts of your mind?

105   Ask Centrum to identify the problematic parts.
Centrum, please identify the part, or parts if there are more than one, of your mind that are actively causing the (problem).

106   Ask Centrum how many parts are actively involved in causing the problem to occur, or in interfering or preventing the goal from being accomplished.
Centrum, how many such parts are active?

107   Ask Centrum to select one of the errant parts, if there is more than one, and establish communications with that part, and to advise you when that has been accomplished.
Centrum, are you in communication with that part?

108   Explain to Centrum that the part is "stuck" in time, aware only of the information available at the time it was formed, and is in ignorance of present reality. Explain Centrum's job as being that of educating the part about present reality, aware of present life situation, values, needs, etc.
Centrum, please communicate with that part in the following way; First, please listen. Find out what the part believes and why it believes what it believes. Then, Centrum, communicate to that part information about present reality. Centrum, that part is stuck in time at that time when it came into being, knowing only what it knew then, in ignorance of your life as it is now. Educate that part, Centrum, about present needs, values and life situation. Persuade that part to your way of thinking.

109   Avoid assuming success. Ask!
Centrum, did you succeed in that task?

110   It is possible that Centrum accomplished more than you requested, or may have identified other active parts.
Centrum, is one or more parts of you mind still active, causing the (problem)?

111   The patient may strongly desire conscious awareness of the work just completed, may be indifferent, or may not want to be aware. Nevertheless, conscious awareness does seem to afford value to the process and, unless there is an expression of conscious opposition, request that Centrum reveal that information to consciousness.
Centrum, please elevate to consciousness awareness of the work you just completed. Please do so by writing it on the chalkboard, by an inner voice, memory, insight or any other means.

112   Express the fact that the real test of completeness of this work is in the real world, yet there is value in finding a way to test it here and now, so that if not complete, we can continue now. Ask the patient to use his or her imagination to project into the future into a situation in which the problem would be expected to manifest. If the patient has difficulty imagining that situation, the work is not complete. Other tests may occur to you. Use them as necessary as an aid in decisions of the moment.

201   It may seem incongruous that Centrum is not aware of what is happening in the patient's life, yet that sometimes occurs, and the patient is usually dysfunctional because of it. Your task is to make Centrum aware of the issue and one way is to ask the patient to verbalize the problem, in simple yet comprehensive terms, after requesting that Centrum listen.

202   At this point in the process, you are dependent upon Centrum. It is necessary that Centrum develop understanding of causal factors and it is your job to facilitate this. It might be that Centrum simply does not understand what is expected, or that Centrum is unable to overcome the blocking of some resistant part, or other issue. By appropriate questions to Centrum, based on your professional sense of the situation, clarify the problem and persuade Centrum to continue with the work.

203   It is possible that Centrum is actively causing the problem that is the focus of treatment, that Centrum disagrees with the conscious opinion of the patient.
Centrum, are you yourself Centrum, are you causing (problem)?

204   Centrum may not understand some aspect of your request, so ask if your request is clear and/or explain in different words. You have requested that Centrum indicate when the task is complete by writing "complete" on the chalkboard, and there has been no response, it may be that you (or the patient) are being impatient and Centrum simply needs more time. Ask Centrum if that is the case.
Centrum, are you involved in the process and need more time? Okay, we will be patient, just let us know by the word "complete" when you have completed the task.

205   You may, or you may not, know how many parts are actually involved causing the presenting problem; you only know there is more than one. Ask Centrum to select one of the parts and to proceed with the protocol. When Centrum has cleared that part, ask Centrum to select another, etc., until all have been cleared.

206   You have requested that Centrum indicate completeness by writing the word "complete" and no response has been forthcoming. Ask Centrum if more time is needed. If no, ask if Centrum is willing to do the work.
Centrum, are you willing to establish communication as I requested?

207   *Centrum, did you succeed in establishing communication with the part, as I requested?*

208   Unconscious entities may deny conscious awareness for reasons of protection of for other reasons that are considered valid. On the other hand, it may be that conscious awareness is not necessary to accomplish the goal. You won't know unless you ask.
Centrum, will conscious awareness be necessary to accomplish the goal?

301   *Centrum, are you willing to continue this work?*

302   You need to know Centrum's opinion, since this is the root of the barrier to the consciously desired change. So, ask. Ask for the opinion to be written, expressed by an inner voice, or other means. When elicited, guide the patient to offer countering views – back and forth – until agreement is reached.

303   In this step, you are seeking a way to encourage communications between the part and Centrum. A fair assumption is that the part is fearful of exposure and this approach has been highly effective in resolving the barrier. *Centrum, is the part willing to consider to information with the provision that it need not expose itself, that it is only required to listen?*

304   A "no" or "no response" to this question will challenge your professional ability to devise an approach that will overcome the barrier. One possible way is to temporarily abandon Subliminal Therapy, perhaps using age-regression techniques to resolve the immediate aspect, and then return to working with Subliminal Therapy. Perhaps request Centrum to select a different part to work with, then come back to this part after requesting the part to listen to the process.

305   *Centrum, please communicate with the part. Inform the part about present life conditions, needs, values and desires. Ensure that the part understands the negative consequences of its influence and persuade the part to support your conscious goals.*

306   Here, the best bet is to assume that the part is, in fact, listening and to ask Centrum to communicate as though that is true. Assume the part is well-intended and appeal to that good intention.
Centrum, please communicate information to this part, information about present life conditions, etc. Be supportive of that part, Centrum, appeal to its good intentions.

307   The part agreed to listen, and apparently has listened to the appeal from Centrum. The next step is to arrange bi-lateral communications between the part and Centrum so that full, mutual understanding can be reached between them.
Centrum, is the part now willing to communicate fully with you in an exchange of positions and opinions?

308   *Centrum, please communicate further information to the part. This time, Centrum, appeal to the positive intention of the part, offer any information you believe may persuade the part to communicate with you.*

309   Being clear that you are asking for the conscious opinion of
        the patient, ask if it is important to him or her to know, at a
        conscious level, about the work just completed. Some will insist
        on knowing, others will not want to know.
        [Patient's name], do you want to know, to understand consciously,
        what Centrum just accomplished?

310   The patient wants to know, and there is value in having that
        knowledge. Therefore, this becomes the focus of therapy. With
        this goal in mind, guide Centrum to eliminate the barrier,
        perhaps by following the basic protocol of Subliminal Therapy.

311   There are many conceivable reasons why Centrum might be
        unwilling to continue. You might be able to anticipate the reason
        and respond effectively, or you might not know the reason. Ask
        if Centrum is willing to reveal the reason for the refusal and use
        this response (if provided) to persuade Centrum.

        Your talents as a clinician will be tested at this juncture. Be
        inventive, knowing that unless Centrum can be persuaded, you
        must shift to another mode of treatment.

Part IV

Applications of Hypnosis

Chapter Thirteen

Applications Having Unique Characteristics

Argue for your limitations,
And sure enough,
They are yours.

Richard Bach (1997)
Illusions

In this chapter, I address a number of applications of hypnosis that I have personally and successfully employed. I offer clinicians my insights and guidance in each case, with the hope that his or her range of use will be expanded. The literature on the applications of hypnosis is voluminous, covering a wide range of problems in the medical domain that are not included here. The reader is referred to the *Journal of the American Society of Clinical Hypnosis* (JASCH) for many such applications.

This chapter is dedicated to listing some of the more typical applications that respond well to hypnotic treatment. In a few instances, I have offered details peculiar to that disorder; however, in most of the applications the following, general procedure can be employed:

1. Establish rapport. This is always essential for success.

2. Educate the patient. Provide the information necessary for that patient, at his or her level of sophistication, to comprehend the procedure you propose to employ. Surprise should never be part of the treatment.

3. Employ hypnosis, suggestively, analytically or in combination, as you deem appropriate.

Academic Applications

Studying

Learning requires perception and understanding of the perceived material; the material must make sense because if it doesn't, it will not be remembered. The focus of attention provided by hypnosis, in combination with suggestions that enhance understanding, can be effective in achieving actual comprehension. The use of the following suggestion, originated by Camilla VanVoorhees, M.D., is preferably read or recited to oneself while in the trance state. It has been found to be of value by undergraduate, medical and law students.

As I now close my eyes and take a deep breath or two, and let it out slowly, I notice a feeling of relaxation flowing through my body.

As I touch my thumb to the ring finger of my right hand, I may feel a special "tingling" sensation spread through my body, permitting ever-greater release of tension and softening of muscles throughout my body.

And, with each breath I release, I can experience yet a little further release of tension, and my mind becomes calmer and less hurried.

Then, focusing my attention on my eyes, I am aware of a different feeling there, no longer responsive in usual ways, reluctant to open, and resisting my efforts to open them, and then refusing to open.

And now I focus my attention on some sound that is present – and the more I focus my attention on that sound, the greater the release of tension within my body and within my mind.

And, while my body feels completely relaxed, and my mind feels at ease, all sounds fade into the background. As I focus my attention on these words, I am ready to consider suggestions of ways in which I can set the stage for learning.

In experiencing these moments of calm contemplation, I am preparing myself – both consciously and unconsciously – for the challenge of learning, and I will find myself challenged by the task.

As I expose myself to the materials being reviewed, my attention will be focused on that material – and other stimuli will remain on the periphery of my awareness, not distracting, not requiring my attention just now.

My attitude toward the challenge of learning will be that of openness to the material reviewed – and, in being open, I will be aware of any detail or any aspect that doesn't quite fit, or that doesn't make sense, and I will seek to understand.

And – in understanding – I will remember.

Also, there in the depth of my mind, will be the ever-present awareness of my developing expectation of passing this course this time *and, with awareness of any reservation, there will be a renewal of my commitment to pass* this time.*"*

Test-taking

It is not uncommon for a student to know the material being tested, yet not be able to competently perform when taking a test on that material. It is as though thoughts and fears of failure interfere with recall, thereby facilitating failure on the test. Given that we are able to consciously attend to only one thought at a time, the possibility of such interference is easily understood; distracting thoughts, fears and conscious struggling to remember preclude communication of the material from memory to consciousness. The question is what to do about it. The answer lies in altering the conditioning imposed by earlier experience, in which the individual learned the unfortunate, limiting patterns of thought.

Just as in so many other issues, the use of hypnosis as an analytical tool is a highly efficient way to alter conditioning. The therapist should guide the individual to use age-regression, Subliminal Therapy, or another analytic hypnotic technique. If Subliminal Therapy is employed, guide the patient to achieve insight, followed by understanding, reframing or re-decision (see Chapter 12). Then follow by asking Centrum to educate the involved unconscious parts about the present life situation, as well as current needs and values, thereby persuading those parts to the position held consciously.

Comprehension and Memory

Many clinicians who employ hypnosis maintain that we mentally record all we perceive, and that, under the right conditions, we have access to those memories. This makes very good sense to me; however, comprehension seems also to be required if we are to remember the material. If we are to learn academic subject matter, we must first perceive it and then comprehend it. If it doesn't make sense to us, i.e., if we do not comprehend it, we will not likely remember it.

Other things, too, may interfere with memory. Even the very struggle to remember something can block the memory. Also, anxiety creates mental tension that may preoccupy our thoughts; depression may preclude rational thought, and fear can elicit concerns that preempt memory. Therefore, the first step in treating memory and/or comprehension problems is to identify the underlying cause of the problem, and it is common that there is no conscious awareness of the genesis of that problem. Subliminal Therapy is by far the most efficient way to identify and resolve such problems.

Accelerated Wound Healing

The mechanics of wound healing involve providing required chemical agents to the wound site over a protracted period. Provision of these agents is accomplished by blood flow to the site; the agents themselves are manufactured in the glands of the body, and the process is controlled by unconscious mentality that is not comprehensible to the conscious mind.

The pattern of the flow of blood in the body is controlled unconsciously. The mechanism of that control is via smooth muscles around the arteries that can constrict, thereby limiting the flow of blood through that artery. By this means, in a situation of "fight or flight," blood is denied to the digestive system, and provided instead to skeletal musculature. Also, through this mechanism, a rich supply of blood can be provided to a wound to promote rapid healing. Moreover, such increased blood flow to a wound site can be created by means of direct hypnotic suggestion. In such cases analysis is not typically required.

Anxiety Treatment

Anxiety is doubtless the most frequently presented problem seen by the helping professions. The symptoms can sometimes be effectively masked pharmacologically; however, treatment is best accomplished psychologically if the disorder is to be resolved and thereby eliminated. In the case of acute, situation-inspired anxiety, cognitive reframing, coupled with reinforcing hypnotic suggestions, may suffice to achieve relief without analytical work. However, in the case of Generalized Anxiety Disorder, two treatment phases are indicated each of which involves training the patient in personal skills. The first addresses the presenting symptoms; the second addresses causal factors.

In the situation of initial contact, it is impressive to both therapist and patient to observe or experience the relief from the symptoms of anxiety (acute or chronic) that are apparent before trance induction. To be sure, the usual rapport-building and information gathering is necessary, although this is often accomplished with difficulty in the face of pressured speech, agitation and distressed demeanor of the patient. However, when the patient is guided to experience trance, the transition from those symptoms to quiet tranquility can border on spectacular. Indeed, the experience of trance is in polar opposition to the experience of anxiety, and just teaching the patient self-hypnosis can be a major step toward resolution.

According to Mark Schucket, M.D., of the UCSD School of Medicine, the roots of generalized anxiety can be consistently traced to one of three causes: A reaction to an ingested substance (including prescriptive medications), a reaction to some physical ailment that has not been recognized consciously, or a reaction to psychological issues. Differentiating among those possibilities may not be straightforward.

- History and discussion of ingested substances shed light; however, this differential diagnosis is probably best defined by eliminating other possibilities. Here are a few substance-related areas to consider:
  - Substance abuse
  - CNS stimulant intoxication
  - CNS depressant withdrawal

- – Sleeping pills
- – Anti-anxiety drugs
- – Alcohol

- • Many medical disorders may not be recognized consciously, hence becoming causal factors, but should be considered, including:
  - – Mitral valve prolapse
  - – Hyperthyroidism
  - – Cardiac disease (e.g., angina, arrhythmias)
  - – Respiratory disease (e.g., chronic obstructive lung disease, pulmonary embolism)
  - – Endocrine disorders (e.g., hypoglycemia, Addison's)
  - – Pernicious anemia
  - – Porphyria
  - – Pheochromocytoma (if accompanied by panic attacks)
  - – Reaction to chronic illness
  - – Arthritis
  - – Asthma
  - – Myocardial infarction
  - – Colitis
  - – Ulcers

- • Identification of existing psychological causes of anxiety is straightforward and is perhaps the preferred first step in the differential diagnosis. Subliminal Therapy is especially efficacious in this regard. If no unconscious elements become apparent in the initial investigation requested of Centrum, the cause of the anxiety is probably not a reaction to psychological issues. If such elements become apparent, resolution is straightforward (see Chapter 12).

Treatment by direct hypnotic suggestions will likely provide at least temporary symptom relief, but when the cause is psychological, and the analytical use of hypnosis is employed, full resolution can be expected. Anything short of full resolution is a strong indication for medical inquiry into unrecognized physical problems.

Acute, psychogenic, recent-onset anxiety can probably be resolved by using hypnosis. Direct symptomatic suggestion coupled with counseling and education will be most efficacious. On the other hand, as mentioned, Generalized Anxiety Disorder will likely require the uncovering of causal influence.

Asthma Treatment

The etiology of asthma has not been well understood; however, there is no question that emotion plays a highly significant role in its exacerbation. Some clinicians conclude that its etiology is psychological, a learned response to certain stimuli that vary from patient to patient. Others conclude its etiology is purely physical, with emotion compounding the problem. In either event, psychological factors are present, and their presence affords psychological, as well as medical, treatment options.

Highly effective psychological treatment of asthma may be accomplished either by the use of direct hypnotic suggestions, which address the symptoms directly, or by analytical techniques that seek to identify causal factors or influences that are significant to its maintenance. In some cases, training in alleviating the symptoms without addressing causal/maintenance factors at all is adequate and effective. This is usually the case when treating children. In other cases, it seems necessary to address the problem analytically, for example, where confronting the symptoms directly does not provide sufficient relief. Descriptions of both approaches to treatment follow.

Relieving the Symptoms of Asthma

Until his death in 1996, Ray LaScolla, M.D., taught a replicable technique of treating asthma to clinicians throughout the country. Some of his lectures were recorded and are available, although he never published his work. The algorithm presented here is derived from such recordings and, in most instances, is a direct reflection of his words. LaScolla did not concern himself with searching for psychological factors; instead he confronted the symptoms directly, teaching hypnotic techniques of muscle relaxation that apply to the smooth muscle systems of the bronchial tree. In this manner, he trained the patient to eliminate the symptoms of asthma by directly influencing the smooth muscle that mediates the symptoms. The technique that is described here is applicable to adults and children alike.

Among professionals who employ hypnosis, there is a lack of agreement about whether this treatment is actually "curative" or only relieves its symptoms. However, they do agree that the subjective experience of the patient can be significantly altered, frequently to the extent that the patient reports a "cure." In any event, as the patient practices the procedure for relief of symptoms, the symptoms occur less frequently.

The objective of the procedure is to achieve relaxation of the smooth muscle systems that occlude the air passageways within the bronchial tree, thus permitting unrestricted passage of air without concerted effort, or the "wheezing" sounds that typically accompany forced breathing.

The LaScolla Procedure:
1.   Guide the patient to experience trance and teach self-hypnosis for future benefit, ensuring adequate depth of trance by using several deepening exercises.

2.   Describe the physical elements involved in an asthma attack by portraying the bronchial system as an inverted tree. Describe the action of smooth muscle to constrict passageways, much as a purse string constricts the opening of the purse, and teach that smooth muscle systems exist in the trunk of the tree (the patient's throat), in its branches, and in its roots as well. Describe the mechanism of the source of the wheezing sound as being the vibration of the air passageways as they become restricted by muscle action.

3.   Call attention to the degree of relaxation now being experi-enced and suggest that such relaxation can be extended into the bronchial tree to relax those muscles, thereby permitting the passageways to open. Give an example, such as: *Just as a rock, held at arms length, will eventually drop to the ground as the muscles of the hand are progressively relaxed, in the same manner, the passageways will open as the smooth muscles relax....*

4.   Ask the patient to deliberately flare his or her nostrils, instructing that this act will be the cue for the release of bronchial muscle tension. Call attention to the sensations experienced as the muscles of the nostrils are alternately relaxed and tightened, with special attention to the feelings of relaxation. Suggest the same physical sensation of relaxation can now be experienced back, up, and into the nasal cavity, as those muscles are relaxed. Ask for, and wait for, an affirmative report of this experience.

5.   Suggest the sensation of relaxation achieved in the nostrils and nasal cavity can be extended, as the relaxation progresses back, into the top of the throat, and then down through the throat (the trunk of the bronchial tree). Ask for, and wait for, an affirmative report of this experience.

6.   Suggest that the relaxation can spread to the right and left sides, where the air passageway divides into the right and left sides of the lungs. Then suggest that the relaxation can continue to spread down into the lungs, as the passageways divide again, and yet again, until even the tiniest passageways are opened, those passageways leading to the air sacs at the inner face of the lungs.

7.   Suggest the patient notice that as the relaxation progresses breathing becomes progressively easier, that it's easier to breathe in, and to breathe out. Suggest that this process of progressive relaxation continue until breathing is effortless and comfortable, "as was true before you ever knew about asthma." Ask for, and wait for, an affirmative report of this experience.

8.   Ask the patient if he or she is willing to demonstrate his or her control of the asthma by bringing on – and then taking away – a mild asthma attack. If necessary, gently persuade the patient to permit this, it being in his or her best interest to learn by experience. When permission is obtained, guide the patient's experience as you offer suggestions for the muscle systems to progressively tighten, beginning in the tiny air sacs and progressing into the larger passageways. And, as this happens, suggest that the patient will notice breathing becoming more effortful. Then, as soon as you observe such labored breathing,

immediately guide the patient to reverse the process, using the flaring of nostrils as the cue, being aware of the sensation of relaxation progressing down through the throat and into the lungs, progressively relaxing the muscles of the "tree," noticing all the while that breathing becomes less effortful and more comfortable with each breath, until it is completely comfortable. Ask for, and wait for, an affirmative report of this experience.

9. Having accomplished the cycle in Step 8, permission to guide the patient to bring on, and then to remove, an attack is again requested – this time to bring on an even more severe attack, this time to the extent of wheezing. Point out that the patient is learning to control the asthma, and that the patient can control it when he or she wishes to do so, in any place, at any time. Repeat the process of Step 8, pointing out that the patient is able to bring on – and then remove – an attack, easily and quickly. By suggestion, guide the "attack" to increase in intensity until both you and the patient are aware of wheezing, and then invite the patient to remove the attack by the use of the cue.

10. Offer suggestions about this new skill becoming a permanent part of the patient's life, to be used at any desired time, and to be quickly and efficiently employed. Request that the patient rouse feeling refreshed, confident, and "good" about himself or herself.

Resolving Causal and/or Maintenance Factors with Subliminal Therapy

The following is a transcription of three one-hour sessions with a patient I will call Jane. The technique employed was analytical, specifically that of Subliminal Therapy, as described in Chapter 12. Unless the reader is familiar with its concepts, the following will not make much sense. The sessions took place in an individual therapy context, with only the therapist and patient present. A single one-hour session of history taking and evaluation preceded these sessions.

Session 1

The patient, Jane, had read my book, *Subliminal Therapy: Utilizing the Unconscious Mind* (Yager, 1985). She was thus familiar with the principles of the technique, and was guided to visualize a chalkboard, upon which Centrum could write as a means of communicating to consciousness. The patient was also instructed to tell me what was written on her chalkboard any time I prefaced my question (or request) with the name "Centrum." Responses from Centrum are capitalized.

Dr.   Centrum, please indicate willingness to communicate by writing the word "yes" on the chalkboard. YES

Dr.   Centrum, are you aware of your conscious concern about the negative effects of the asthma? YES

Dr.   Centrum, are you willing to cooperate, to work, as I guide and teach you how, toward the goal of eliminating the asthma? YES

Dr.   Centrum, do you have the ability to communicate with other parts of the mind and to access memories? YES

Dr.   Centrum, please use those abilities to investigate the cause and development of the asthma. Review whatever information is available to you about its history, from the first experience to the present. Communicate with other parts of the mind that are involved and review available memories. Then let us know when you have done so by writing the word "complete" on the chalkboard. COMPLETE

Dr.   Centrum, do you now understand how and when the asthma came into existence and why it has continued to be a part of your life? YES

Dr.   Centrum, is the asthma serving a useful purpose in your life now? YES

Dr.   Centrum, is it okay for you to have conscious awareness of the purpose being served now? YES

Dr.   Centrum, please elevate that awareness to consciousness now, by whatever means are appropriate, by writing on the chalkboard, by an inner voice, by memory, or by other means. Jane, please let me know when you have that awareness consciously.

Jane   I'm having some memories of six years ago. I'm somewhere I don't want to be. I'm feeling trapped/suffocated/anxious. I don't know what to do. The words "SIGNALS ANXIETY" are written on the chalkboard.

Dr.   Jane, what is your conscious opinion about the meaning of all that?

Jane   I don't need such an extreme signal (the asthma) to know something is bothering me!

Dr.   Does it make sense to you consciously/logically that you would have learned to respond as you did in that situation?

Jane   Yes, it makes sense.

Dr.   Centrum, do you agree you learned to experience asthma in that situation and that you don't need the asthma anymore? NO

Dr.   Centrum, do you believe you still need the asthma as a signal of some kind? YES

Dr.   Jane, you have spontaneously slipped into trance, and that's fine. Now I ask that you rouse yourself, so we can talk about what has happened.

Jane   (Tearfully) I don't *want* to have asthma anymore!

Dr.   Jane, you can interact with Centrum yourself, without my assistance and guidance. Please practice that now, communicate with Centrum to learn whatever you need to know about the beginnings of the asthma, and say what you need to say to persuade Centrum to your point of view – that is, that you don't need the asthma in your life now, even though you may have considered it necessary at some time in the past. When you have completed that discussion, let me know.

Jane   OK, I think everything is all right now. I made a promise to run if I feel trapped again.

Dr.   Centrum, is it okay for you to be free of the asthma under the condition that you run as agreed? YES

Dr.   Centrum, how many parts of your mind were actively involved in causing the asthma? THREE

Dr.   Centrum, are you in communication with all three? YES

Dr.   Centrum, are all three parts now in agreement with you, and your conscious opinion, about the asthma no longer being necessary or desirable? NO

Dr.   Centrum, how many of the parts are not in agreement? ONE

Dr.   Centrum, please communicate with that part to learn why it still disagrees. COMPLETE

Dr.   Centrum, do you now understand the basis of its belief? YES

Dr.   Centrum, do you agree with the position held by the part? NO

Dr.   Centrum, do you agree with your consciously held position that the asthma is no longer necessary? YES

Dr.   Centrum, please communicate further with that part to insure it is given the information you now have, information that has persuaded you to your way of thinking about the asthma. Centrum, that part is acting in your best interest, as it understands your best interest. It is acting on the basis of what *was* at some time in the past, in ignorance of your present life situation. Educate that part, Centrum. Persuade that part to your way of thinking and let us know by the word "complete" when you have done so. COMPLETE

Dr. Centrum, were you successful? YES

Dr. Centrum, are all parts of your mind *now* in agreement that the asthma is no longer necessary and can be eliminated? YES

Dr. Jane, please rouse yourself again.

> *Note: The patient was then guided to experience trance and suggestions were given for clearing her nasal cavity – that it become clear and dry and comfortable. After clearing was completed, an experience that surprised the patient, the session ended.*

Session 2 (Six days later)

The patient came to the session reporting a "bad" week. She had been very symptomatic, almost having to go to the emergency room on two occasions. She had kept her end of the bargain with Centrum, but had not been able to communicate with Centrum as she had during the last session. She came into the session symptomatic, with audible "wheezing" sounds emanating from her chest.

Dr. Centrum, are you aware the asthma has continued in force? YES

Dr. Centrum, do you understand why? YES

Dr. Centrum, would it be okay for you to understand why at a conscious level? NO

Dr. Centrum, would it be okay for you to reveal the reason/s to me without there being conscious memory of what is revealed? YES

Dr. Centrum, please reveal the reasons without conscious memory. CAN'T – CONSCIOUS IS AWARE

Dr. Centrum, do you now (again) believe the asthma is serving useful purpose? YES

Dr. Centrum, is that purpose the "signaling of anxiety," as came up last time? NO

Dr. Centrum, are you "protecting" Jane by denying conscious awareness of the reason? NO

Dr. Centrum, would it be okay for you to know, consciously, the reason for denying access? IT WOULD REVEAL TOO MUCH

Dr. Centrum, is it necessary for you to experience the asthma symptoms as often, or as intensely, as you have during the past week? IT IS NOT

Dr. Centrum, is there some reason for you having experienced those symptoms this past week? REMINDER

Dr. Centrum, reminder of what? NOT PROTECTION, SELF-PUNISHMENT

Dr. Centrum, are you punishing yourself by causing the asthma? YES

Dr. Centrum, is there conscious awareness of what you are being punished for? NO

Dr. Centrum, what, then, can possibly be accomplished by causing punishment? NOTHING

Dr. Centrum, is it okay for you to have conscious awareness of only "why" the punishment? OKAY

Dr. Centrum, please provide that awareness now.

Jane It was punishment for "self-perfectionism ways."

Dr.   Centrum, is that accurate? YES

Dr.   Jane, do you consciously understand what is going on?

Jane   I'm trying to.

Dr.   Jane, what is your best guess at this time?

Jane   I never saw myself that way. My mother is very perfectionistic and I don't want to be that way!

Dr.   Centrum, do you support that conscious position just expressed? YES

Dr.   Centrum, how does punishment serve any useful purpose in that light? IT DOESN'T

Dr.   Centrum, are you now willing to stop causing the asthma, to reverse that pattern? YES

Dr.   Centrum, are you capable of *stopping* the asthma symptoms? YES

Dr.   Centrum, please take whatever steps are necessary to do that now and let us know when you have done so. COMPLETE

Dr.   Centrum, is there yet another part of the mind involved, another dynamic in the picture, anything that might cause the asthma to continue? NO

Dr.   Centrum, do you now have conscious awareness of all of the dynamics involved? YES

Dr.   Centrum, thank you for your cooperation. Are you willing to continue to communicate with consciousness? YES

Dr.   Jane, please rouse yourself from trance and let's talk about things.

Jane   The wheezing is gone! The biggest test will be when I laugh.

> *Note: At this point, I trained the patient in the asthma elimination technique taught by LaScolla, as described in preceding paragraphs.*

Session 3 (Seven days later)

The patient reported a reduction in frequency of asthma attacks from two-to-three per day to only two during the past week, and that she was successful in stopping the attacks on both occasions by employing the LaScolla technique. She also reported her "allergies" had continued to bother her and, since a connection between asthma and allergies is frequently reported, we decided to address the allergies as well.

Dr.   Centrum, are you aware of the allergic reactions you have been experiencing? YES

Dr.   Centrum, are you willing to cooperate, as in the past, in an effort to eliminate them? YES

Dr.   Centrum, please investigate the roots of the allergies. Review memories and communicate with other parts of the mind that are involved to learn whatever can be learned about the how, when, and where of its beginning, and why it has continued to be a part of your life. Let us know when you have completed that task. COMPLETE

Dr.   Centrum, do you believe you now understand the etiology, the cause, of the allergies? No response

Dr.   Centrum, how old were you when the allergies began? VERY YOUNG

Dr.   Centrum, was it before you learned to walk? YES

Dr.   Centrum, do you believe the allergies are psychogenic, that their cause is psychological, rather than purely physical? YES

Dr.   Centrum, will it be okay for you to consciously remember the experiences that prompted those reactions? YES

Dr.   Centrum, please bring those memories to consciousness now. Jane, just be curious to see what comes to your mind, then share with me whatever you are willing to share.

> *Note: Almost half an hour of narration by Jane followed, disclosing a confusing experience as an infant in the presence of quarreling parents. She was aware of what happened, of her emotional reaction at the time, of her physical reaction at the time, and she was able to clearly identify the ongoing influence of the event in the form of her allergies. She concluded the allergies were a purely conditioned response she no longer needs or wants.*

Dr.   Centrum, do you agree with your conscious conclusion that the allergies are no longer needed or wanted? YES

Dr.   Centrum, does any part of your mind, for any reason whatsoever, want the allergies to continue? NO

Dr.   Centrum, as a matter of my personal curiosity, why did you not respond to my question minutes ago about your understanding of the etiology of the allergies? ORIGINS WERE COMING TO HER BUT WEREN'T CLEAR

Dr.   Centrum, thank you for your cooperation. Please continue to influence your life in such way that asthma and allergies can be avoided.

> *Note: Three weeks after the last session, the patient reported she had had no asthma attacks, and no use of her inhaler or medications, since that time. She also volunteered her opinion that the asthma had been triggered by her allergic reactions and that she had been only minimally bothered by her allergies.*

Breast Enlargement

At first glance, it would seem wildly improbable that breast size could be influenced by mental activity, yet that seems to be the case. Although I know of no studies involving breast reduction, there have been a number of studies in which increased breast size was accomplished (Erickson, 1960; Staib & Logan, 1997; Willard, 1977), and one doctoral dissertation studied the phenomenon (Nyquist, 1986). My patients have succeeded in the few cases I have worked with, following the guidelines of the ASCH studies, with the additional use of Subliminal Therapy to identify and resolve mental barriers to increased breast size.

I shall make no statements regarding possible mechanisms for mental influence on the development of physical tissue, leaving that to medical research or to the imagination of the reader. Rather, I will wonder about the cellular construction of the breast and the cellular construction of those growths (malignant or not) that have reportedly been reduced or eliminated by suggestion.

I employ the following steps in training a patient to enlarge her breasts:

1. I will ensure that that patient has the assistance necessary to measure her breast size on a weekly basis. Consistent posture at the time of each measurement is essential. In a standing position, with arms extended horizontally from her sides, three measures are taken: circumferential, nipple-to-nipple across the front, and nipple-to-nipple around the back of the neck. Just as in the case of weight reduction protocols, the frequent reinforcement of progress is important, at least, and possibly essential.

2. She is trained in the self-use of hypnosis, including the experience of phenomena that validate trance to her satisfaction.

3. While in trance, I will guide her to focus her attention on her breasts, aware of whatever sensations she is experiencing in her breasts. Then I offer the following suggestion: *"As you continue to focus your attention on your breasts, notice as a sense of warmth forms and increases in your breasts – a pleasant sense as the*

warmth increases. Let me know when that feeling of warmth is clear and distinct." I will then repeat suggestions until the feeling of warmth is reported.

4. While she continues to experience the feeling of warmth, I will offer the following, additional suggestions: *"As the warmth continues, there in your breasts, use your imagination in this way: Imagine an increase in blood flow into your breasts, bringing the nutrients and chemical stimulants that are necessary to encourage cellular growth. Of course, the warmth you are feeling is actually there because of an increase in blood flow. Now, by imagining the flow of nutrients and other agents, the cells of your breasts multiply and grow to multiply again and again. And, as the cells grow and multiply, your breasts swell and enlarge, becoming full and firm, just the way you want them to be."*

5. The patient is instructed to repeat the self-induction, followed by the imagery of the training experience, as frequently as conditions permit, at least on a daily basis. She is then followed on a weekly basis.

Criminal Investigation

That hypnosis is of marked value in the law enforcement investigative setting is no longer contested. Witnesses to crimes are often interviewed while in trance, with frequent substantive increases in both the quantity and accuracy of the information obtained. However, in some states legislation prohibits, or case law has evolved that prohibits, the use of hypnotically refreshed memories in criminal trial procedures. In some states, law enforcement must therefore "sacrifice" witnesses who are interviewed under hypnosis, balancing the investigative value of potential information with the value the witness might have on the witness stand.

A pertinent question is whether *any* witness in an interview situation can avoid experiencing hypnosis, even though no formal induction has been accomplished. The answer, of course, depends upon one's definition of hypnosis. We may someday arrive at a generally agreed upon definition of hypnosis; however, I do not expect it in my lifetime. All efforts to measure or even to quantify the state have been unconvincing, leaving the law, clinician, and researcher with subjective judgment as the only available measure. True, there are indicators that an individual is experiencing hypnosis, such as muscular relaxation and calm, stillness of the body, yet, there are many exceptions to these indicators as well. The observation of an individual being interviewed in a situation that is subjectively perceived as pressured will consistently reveal several of the "signs" associated with the hypnotic experience. By these criteria, any witness who is interviewed, with or without hypnosis, should be excluded from testifying in court.

Those who claim hypnotically refreshed memory must not be admitted in court point out that such testimony might be confabulated or distorted by any of several factors. They are correct! However, what they say applies to non-hypnotically refreshed memory as well. Dywan and Bowers (1983), Pettinati (1988) and Stalnaker and Riddle (1932) all affirm that hypnosis increases recall of *both* correct *and* incorrect material. If memories are formed consisting of the data *as perceived* by the subject, then such memories would be subject to error in perception, regardless of the retrieval method used.

The oft-staged academic experiment in which a disruption of usual classroom procedure is accomplished by having a stranger run into the room, execute several unexpected behaviors and run out again, graphically illustrates the phenomenon of inaccurate recall. When class members are separately questioned about the event, as many different stories are obtained as there are members of the class. Are the differences accountable by different perceptions, emotional states, encoding mechanisms, recall mechanisms, or other confounding variables? We do not know. Yet, we would not preclude those witnesses from testifying in a court of law. Kroger and Douce (1979) make the point that: "Recall may be distorted by method or may be inaccurate or misleading, drawbacks that also exist at non-hypnotic levels."

Precluding hypnotically refreshed memory from the courtroom is premature; we need to know more about the mechanisms of memory, encoding, accessing and retrieval, before we disallow such a potentially rich resource.

It seems entirely possible that hypnosis, properly employed, facilitates *accuracy* of memory by reducing anxiety, releasing inhibition, and facilitating access to unconsciously stored material. Perhaps our emphasis on the *inaccuracy* of hypermnesia is misdirected and research emphasis should now be placed on identifying what is *accurate*.

Q & A Regarding Hypnosis and Memory

Is hypnosis actually an aid in remembering? Yes! The reader is referred to Chapter 4 for a discussion of the subject.

Why can't people just remember? We all experience memory loss. As an example, we sometimes awaken with the memory of the dream we just had, fresh and vivid and in Technicolor, and then a few seconds later we know we had a dream, but darned if we can remember what it was all about. Also, it seems that we may sometimes unconsciously choose not to remember, perhaps because it would be unpleasant, frightening or threatening in some way. And, in a state of excitement or trauma, we may focus our conscious attention on someone or something and then, through peripheral awareness, record additional information in memory, information that is not consciously recognized at the time. Depending on several variables, using hypnosis appropriately can permit the bypass of such unconscious barriers, and may permit a clearer memory of the event in question, with opportunity to examine, even in slow motion, details not recognized before.

Can hypnosis be used as a truth serum? No. A person can lie while in a hypnotic trance just as proficiently as at any other time.

Why are the courts so sensitive about the use of hypnosis? They are sensitive because of the possibility the investigator using hypnosis might, intentionally or otherwise, interject ideas or distort the memory of the witness during hypnosis. However, the states are not in agreement on the regulation of its use. According to Paul Kincade, one of our better-informed advocates of forensic hypnosis, the states break down as follows:

Hypnotically Refreshed Memories	Number of States
Admissible in all cases	5
Inadmissible in all cases	3
Safeguarded	12
Pre-hypnosis statements admitted	21
Not regulated	9

Only California, Nevada, Oregon, Texas, Washington, and the District of Columbia have legislation regulating its use; all other states that regulate its use do so by case law. Also, in all instances, there are no restrictions on the use of hypnosis by a *defendant* in a criminal case; the right of the defendant to use hypnosis is guaranteed by the U.S. Constitution. Nor is its use restricted in civil cases. The most recent reversal of this policy was accomplished in Nevada, where Statute 48.039 was passed in 1997, permitting the unrestricted use of hypnosis by trained police officers. This statute, authored by Paul Kincade, stands as a model for other states.

With respect to the Federal Courts, the U.S. Supreme Court ruling in Daubert *v.* Merrell Dow Pharmaceuticals in 1993, removed the last barrier to the use of hypnosis in criminal cases in Federal Courts. Federal investigators are now free to use hypnosis without hesitation, although specific guidelines must be followed.

What is the Law in California?

The California legislature has set the example for the other states, except for Nevada and Texas, and was one of the first to pass legislation regulating hypnotically refreshed memory. I have used the California experience to demonstrate the process by which such regulations are established. The California Supreme Court has approved the use of hypnosis in criminal proceedings, as long as it is understood that a witness cannot testify as to material recovered via hypnosis. This approval was contained in the opinion rendered in the case of People *v.* Shirley (31 Cal. 3d 18, 1982). In response to Shirley, the Legislature enacted Section 795 of the California Evidence Code in 1984 to formally regulate the use of hypnosis. The section was then amended in 1987 to recognize the right of a defendant to use hypnosis in his or her own defense and, in doing so, inadvertently created a discriminatory double standard that penalizes the honest citizen by presuming hypnosis to be reliable for the defendant, but not for the victim.

Section 795 provides specific conditions under which testimony of *pre-hypnosis* memories may be admitted in a criminal matter, even though the witness has experienced hypnosis for investigative purposes. Such testimony, however, may only pertain to memories that were available *before* the hypnotic experience. To accomplish this condition, Section 795 provides for full, formal disclosure of information remembered before hypnosis is employed, and further specifies the conditions of that hypnotic interview. These conditions include: the interview must be conducted by a licensed clinician; no members of the law enforcement personnel, the defense, or the prosecution may be present; and the interview must be video and audio recorded.

Under the provisions of Section 795, Stage 1 of the interview consists of a pre-hypnotic period of statements by the witness, and responses to questions posed to the witness, relating to the incident in question. Only this information will hereafter be admissible in court. Stage 2 consists of the induction of trance. Stage 3 consists of the hypnotic interview, which will probably again cover the previous information, and will also include probing questions and guided review of the circumstances from different perspectives.

Do the limits of Section 795 of the Evidence Code apply to defendants? No. The consequence of this legislation has been to raise the specter of hypnotically refreshed memory being accepted as reliable for the defendant and not for the victim or witness. There are no restrictions on the use of hypnosis as an aid in the defense of an individual.

What advantage does Section 795 offer the police investigator? As limited by Shirley, without the provisions of Section 795, any witness who had experienced hypnosis as an aid in investigation would be prohibited from *all* testimony at trial. With Section 795, at least the pre-hypnosis memories are admissible, and the investigator is free to seek additional investigative clues via the hypnotic interview.

If the investigator is not permitted to be present, how can progressive questions be posed? It is generally true that clinicians are not trained in investigative questioning and involvement of the investigator is indicated. Fortunately, communications from the investigator *to the clinician* during the interview are not precluded. Thus, the investigator can be watching and listening electronically and feeding questions to the clinician by means not perceived by the witness, e.g., via an earphone or written notes.

If law enforcement cannot be present, how can we use police artists and IdentiKits? Assuming the images recalled during the hypnotic experience are clear, and assuming appropriate guidance, they will be remembered after the hypnotic session is complete. Thus, the use of artists and IdentiKits will be possible after the session. The Nevada Statute provides for the presence of a composite artist during the hypnotic interview and, in the case of a minor, a parent or guardian.

What if the witness is not required for testimonial purposes? If the witness is not considered essential for testimony in court, the investigator is free to employ hypnosis as desired, of course assuming the witness is agreeable. This situation might occur when there are multiple witnesses to a crime, for example.

Are there legitimate reasons for not using hypnosis, even with all the safeguards of 795? Certainly. The prosecutor may be concerned about the jury's reaction to hypnosis, or, if the witness is not too sharp mentally, believe the witness could be discredited by the defense. It is clearly necessary for law enforcement to cooperate with the prosecutor. Moreover, if some important bit of information is sought, such as a license number, the color of a shirt, or who was standing where, the value obtained may be worth "throwing away" a witness by interacting hypnotically outside the restrictions of Section 795.

Dental Applications

As is true in all clinical situations, the patient's mental state is foremost in impacting the subjective experience of dental problems, as well as procedures.

Anxiety

Aside from the subjective distress experienced by the patient, anxiety also results in muscular tension that can inhibit treatment by restricting the degree to which the patient can open his or her mouth, and defensive, physical reactions, such as heart palpitations, can interfere and may result in the patient not seeking treatment at all. The treatment of anxiety is covered earlier in this chapter.

Bruxing

Bruxing is the unconscious gnashing or grinding of the teeth, often with consequent structural damage. Although typically taking place while asleep, it may also occur during waking hours, even with conscious awareness, but without conscious ability to stop the behavior. In the event there is waking bruxing, there is a high probability of nocturnal bruxing as well. As with other compulsive disorders, it is the consequence of prior conditioning and can be resolved by using hypnosis analytically.

Extractions

To my knowledge, only anecdotal reports of reducing the force required to extract a tooth by means of hypnotic suggestion exist; however, if true, such use would be of significant benefit to both dentist and patient. In any event, a relaxed patient does better overall.

Gagging

The gag reflex can be stimulated by physical contact with the uvula and other areas in the mouth and throat, by emotions, certain tastes, suggestions, and by imagined events. Since its fundamental function is to enhance survival, it is not easily defeated; yet, in trance, the reflex can be substantially subdued by suggestion. Just by being guided to experience trance, without other formal procedures, the patient may be able to comfortably tolerate necessary procedures. Through the use of hypnotic analysis, the incidence of hyper-gagging in reaction to expectation (i.e., imagined events) may be eliminated altogether, thus reducing trauma for the patient and easing the life of the dentist.

Post-treatment Pain

The reported duration of discomfort following dental treatments varies greatly. For example, a root canal may disable one patient for multiple days, whereas another returns to work immediately following the procedure. Expectation seems to be the key element in determining duration. To the degree hypnosis can influence expectation, it can control post-treatment discomfort and, since suggestions cost so little, and the risk is near nonexistent, we should use them.

Dissociative Disorders

Hypnosis is considered by some authorities to be a dissociative phenomenon, probably based on the ability of the subject to consciously dissociate from emotional experience, yet emotion may also be experienced at an unconscious level, even without conscious awareness.

Our ability to dissociate is universally, and often unconsciously, employed as a defense against unwelcome thoughts and experiences; it is only when the process becomes dysfunctional that the clinician is consulted. Since dissociation can be inspired or impaired by suggestion, treatment of the disorder is facilitated by the use of direct suggestions, as well as analytic hypnotic techniques.

Fugue, Sensory Alterations and Dissociative Disorder NOS

In the treatment of fugue states, sensory alterations (*e.g.*, blindness or deafness) and Dissociative Disorder NOS, direct suggestive techniques are apt to be effective. Such suggestions, coupled with information relating the suggestion to rational consideration of current issues and status, may inspire dramatic change. For example, if psychogenic blindness is the objective of treatment, this suggestion, while in trance, may be effective: *"It will be okay for you to see my hand, now, in this situation, to ensure your eyes are in fact functioning as they should. It will be okay, now, for you to see my hand, because, as a mature adult, you understand the importance of being able to do so. Now, while staying in trance, open your eyes and see my hand, there, in front of you."* If it is necessary to define *why* the blindness occurred, it will be necessary to use hypnosis analytically.

Multiple Personality Disorder = Dissociative Identity Disorder

In the case of Dissociative Identity Disorder (DID), which is considered the ultimate dissociative disorder, hypnosis is useful in establishing communication *with* alter personalities, in establishing communication *between* alter personalities, and in bringing about the integration *of* the alter personalities. Outlines of effective procedures follow.

Though the ideal objective in the treatment of DID is total integration of all alter personalities, so that the individual is able to function normally in all respects, the achievable goal often becomes a compromise. One or more alter personalities may take an arbitrary, non-negotiable stand and refuse to integrate with the others. In such cases, the goal becomes that of negotiating the highest level of functioning possible for the person and, in general, great improvement is achievable. The clinician who decides to work with this population is advised to do so with full awareness that treatment will be extensive and progress will probably be slow; sessions may extend over many months. Nevertheless, the work is fulfilling to the clinician.

Treatment of patients with DID differs from the treatment of normal individuals in that effective functioning of normal individuals is possible by virtue of the integrated functioning of mental capacities, each the product of past experience. In this "normal" situation, the lessons of past experience are brought to the forefront of decision-making on a continuing basis, and modified by further experience, rather than being maintained in isolation. In the case of

DID, alter personalities seem to be made up of multiple influences that originated in the course of life experiences and then became isolated from other experiences. A plausible explanation for the establishment of an alter personality is that when an individual is in a situation where he or she is actually unable to cope, the person may mentally vacate the situation, leaving a void in which a new personality is formed, a personality with all of the characteristics associated with that new situation.

Establishing communication *with* alter personalities

People who are troubled by multiple personalities are usually highly intelligent, but disorganized and socially dysfunctional. They are commonly not able to maintain employment or social relationships, and they are often destitute. It is difficult to imagine what it would be like to find ourselves in an unknown place, not knowing how we got there, or to be accused of things we know full well we did not do, or to find ourselves in trouble without knowing why. This is the plight of those with this disorder. At the beginning of treatment, the "host" personality is probably unable to contact the alter personalities, and may not even know of their existence.

The first task in treating this disorder is to identify the alter personalities, and hypnosis is of essential value in accomplishing this task. I teach the host personality how to go into trance, and repeat that trance induction multiple times, so the state is easily accomplished. Then, I take advantage of that characteristic of trance that facilitates the response of alter personalities to my request to "come out," to "assume dominance at this time, in this place." Responses to my requests are immediate, and I am often surprised by the interactions that occur with them. I find they will cooperate, and will be forthcoming about their purpose and function, together with their own beliefs, values, and opinions. The personalities will probably already have names; however, if not, they should be asked to give themselves names for logistical purposes. The number of alters may range from two to 100 or more and, if the number is large, I am concerned only with the dominant ones, those who emerge most often, and who have the greatest impact on the patient's life. The age range of alters can span from less than a year to adulthood.

I learn as much as I can about each of the "alters," as this information may be necessary when I begin the process of integration.

I focus my efforts on identifying the intent or purpose of each of
the alters. Initially, one alter or more may profess determination to
execute self-injury and may, in fact, succeed in self-mutilation to
some degree. Such a position is usually aimed at self-punishment
for some past behavior that is unconsciously seen as "bad," even
though it is apparent to the host personality that the guilt is not
justified. Even in this case the behavior can be reframed as being
positively motivated, and having thus joined with the offending
alter, communication is facilitated and rational thought can generally be instituted to achieve cooperation by that alter.

Establishing communication *between* alter personalities
Just as the host personality may not have knowledge of the existence of one or more of the alter personalities, so the alters may not
have knowledge of one another. The first task of the clinician is
to develop such awareness, and then encourage communication
between them. In this way, their common interests can be identified
and cooperative efforts effected, thus enabling improved functioning of the individual. This is also a preparatory step of "stage-setting" for their integration. Awareness of one alter by another may
be engineered by confronting the one with the fact of the "effects"
of another; for example, while communicating with one, directing
attention to a behavior that is present, even while the first is dominant. Then it can be pointed out that another influence – possibly
another personality – is causing that irrational behavior.

To facilitate communication between the alters, consent of both
must first be obtained and a vehicle of such communication be
identified. Such a vehicle might first be a chalkboard, or perhaps
each is encouraged to listen for an inner voice, which will be the
voice of the other.

Engineering integration *of* alter personalities
Integration of the alter personalities is accomplished in two steps:
First, the alter personalities are persuaded by logical reasoning that
it is in their best interest, and the best interest of the individual,

that they join together, abandoning their individual characteristics and supporting the common good (a step that may require many sessions); second, actual integration is accomplished by means of an imagined ceremony.

Persuasion is accomplished by slow, patient education of the alters by the clinician. By reframing the positive intention of the alters, no matter how negative they may initially appear, they are individually led by rational reasoning to the conclusion that integration is advisable. In accomplishing this, the clinician must interact with very young and with older alters, as well as with compliant and defiant ones. In each case, the needs of that alter must be acknowledged and accommodated in the process of being educated about current reality.

The *ceremony* in which the alters are joined together is enacted in the imagination of the patient. The ceremony may be designed and created by the clinician or by the patient. A typical ceremony might include the image of merging clouds, or the blending of different colored, fluid streams, each representing one of the alters, or it might be a formal ceremony. The duration of the ceremony is best left up to the patient, the clinician being outside the process insofar as is possible.

Once integrated, stability can be expected; only further trauma will fragment the common personality that has emerged. Requests for the emergence of independent alters, integrated while in trance, will not usually be acted upon. It is as though the alters have ceased to exist as independent entities.

Although I have been treating MPD for many years using hypnosis, I have only recently begun to use Subliminal Therapy with these patients. It has proven to be surprisingly effective. Just as with other patients, Centrum appears to be both reliable and cooperative in accomplishing all of the steps required to achieve integration.

Grief

I am indebted to the work of Edgar Jackson (1947), whose book, *Understanding Grief*, inspired the protocol that follows. In it, he defined the elements of the process of working through grief; I amended that protocol to conform to hypnotic procedures. As envisioned, working through grief involves transferring mental energy from awareness of the past to awareness of the present, with consideration for the future. The procedure has been of great value to many of my patients, permitting normal functioning immediately following the procedure.

In a very real sense, the loss that is grieved marks the beginning of a new life for the individual. Many changes in the individual's life have just occurred, and the work required is that of identifying those changes and preparing for the new life by accommodating those changes. This is the essence of working through grief, and trance can greatly facilitate the process. By using the procedure that follows, a motivated, grieving patient can work through grief in an hour or so; the days, weeks, or months usually required for the grieving process are unnecessary.

If the loss is recent and severe, such as the death of a close family member, it may be days or weeks before the patient is ready for the process outlined below. In the interim, calming the patient during episodes of intense grief by simply listening, by making physical contact in an appropriate way, such a holding his or her hand, or placing your hand on his or her shoulder, or by offering communications that you care and will do all a therapist can do. When the person has regained composure and is able to rationally consider his or her status, the therapist should utilize the following steps with the patient in a trance state:

Note:

> For illustration purposes, I refer to a case in which a woman has lost her spouse.

The following steps are presented in the form of recommended instructions for the clinician's use.

1. After introducing the concept of transferring mental energy from the past to the future, and the concept of a new life beginning with the loss of her spouse, guide her to experience trance. Then, while in trance, ask the patient to silently review the relationship with the spouse, from the beginning of the relationship to the present, to obtain an overall perspective of that relationship, defining the most important events and experiences.

2. The emotional reactions the patient is experiencing in the present can be identified through respectful, considerate queries. A sense of loss may be accompanied by feelings of anger, guilt, or fear. The patient should be assured that all of these responses are appropriate and understandable.

3. If guilt is expressed, the basis for it should be determined. Perhaps there were things she should have done but did not do, or things she should not have done but did. Self-forgiveness will be required in this case. If there is anger, she can be guided to forgive the offending party – not for the sake of the offender, but for her own sake. If there is fear, a clear definition of what is feared must be derived. The patient should then be guided to rationally confront that fear, making appropriate decisions about its degree and clarifying options along the way.

4. The next step is to guide her to identify the needs her spouse was satisfying in her life, and patiently ensure that she has identified multiple, possible ways to satisfy each of those needs.

5. The "key" people, who are going to form the basis of the new life, the life that began upon her husband's death, must now be identified. These are the persons who will satisfy those needs he had been satisfying, whether material, emotional, or otherwise.

6. Guide her to identify the new problems she can anticipate encountering in this new life, and then to consider multiple, possible ways to solve each of those problems.

7. New responsibilities should be identified, as well as any barriers to her fulfilling those responsibilities.

8. She should be guided to consider the lessons she learned from her spouse, noting that his influence will continue in this and in other ways for as long as she lives – and probably beyond that, through her influence on others.

9. She should also be asked what her husband would have wanted for her. Would he have wanted her to grieve endlessly, be disabled by grief, and perhaps cause others distress as well?

10. The patient should then be guided to identify any other positive influence that continues, rejoicing in each such influence.

11. Finally, the patient should be guided to create her sanctuary, as described in Chapter 9. Point out that she is in *total* control of *everything*, and suggest that she bring him to her, there in that sanctuary, where she can say anything she needs to say, and hear anything she needs to hear. When she has indicated completion, it should be suggested that she say goodbye, letting her husband go his way, sending him with her love and her caring, knowing she can again be with him there in that sanctuary whenever she wishes.

Gynecological Applications

Infertility

Infertility can sometimes be explained by the existence of medical problems. However, sometimes all medical workups of both partners are negative, and the woman still does not conceive. Is it possible that mental influence can interfere with conception?

Logic, plus clinical experience, tells me such influence is possible. After all, if emotions can impact glandular activity, interfere with digestive process, and cause hypertension, why should the reproductive process be exempt from such influence?

Although my clinical experience is limited in this area, and very few (even anecdotal) reports are available in the literature, those cases in my practice in which the woman has become pregnant after having resolved psychological issues that were apparently preventing conception have impressed me.

Obstetrical Applications

This area is worthy of an entire book; however, only superficial consideration is possible here. As in all areas of medical practice, emotions are a primary source of influence on physical condition; however, that is particularly true in this area. From the process of birthing to correction of menstrual abnormalities and from menopausal considerations to infertility, it is important to ensure balance in mental perspectives and functioning. Hypnosis is the intervention of choice for these purposes.

Morning Sickness Relief

Not all newly pregnant women experience morning sickness; however, it is experienced by most to some degree. Considering the onslaught of realizations the woman is facing, it is surprising that more women do not have this reaction, or do not have it more intensely than they do.

For the woman, pregnancy generally means nine months of absolute involvement, focused relentlessly on concerns about personal needs and at the same time limited in the ability to fulfill those needs. It means her life is committed for at least the next 18 years. It may also mean agonizing concern about the perfection of the baby to be born. All of this, most often coupled with fear of the delivery process, can clearly be expected to engender a reaction, and what more normal reaction can be imagined than voiding the "physical problem." Of course, the physical problem is in the uterus, not in the stomach, so throwing up achieves nothing but further distress. The point is that, barring abnormal medical complications, the etiology of morning sickness is probably psychological.

There are, of course, many competing theories about morning sickness, with medical experts maintaining it to be a consequence of hormonal imbalance. If correct, one wonders how the elimination of the problem using hypnotic treatment can be explained.

Treatment

Treatment of morning sickness requires taking a thorough history and inquiry into intensely personal information at a level not possible without fully developed rapport between patient and professional. Not only is the history of the pregnancy required, but also a history of relevant relationships, marital status, the condition of that relationship, available ego-support, core values, and sources of stress.

Does the woman want the pregnancy? Does she want a baby at all? Does the father want a baby? Is the relationship with the father stable in her view? Is there a possible question about paternity? Is there concern about her health or her medical history? How fearful is she about the delivery? Is she naïve about the course of her pregnancy, or is she well informed? Is she considering abortion? The answers to such questions are essential, and problematic issues must be recognized and appropriate decisions made. Finally, there may be issues not recognized consciously, issues that nevertheless prompt the reaction of morning sickness. It is advisable to inquire about unconscious issues by means of ideomotor response, or by more formal approaches such as Subliminal Therapy. Failure to identify the true, underlying issues guarantees failure in relieving distress.

As in most treatment situations, it is my practice to begin therapy by teaching the patient self-hypnosis. Not only does this provide her with a skill she can use to quell the upsurges of nausea on her own, it also provides relief from nausea while we work together, and facilitates investigation into causal issues.

Next, information about possible psychogenesis is imparted, and it is pointed out that vomiting is a normal reaction when unwelcome or irritating substances are ingested, that the autonomic nervous system becomes involved in executing even unconscious stimuli, and that this is an example of physical reactions to emotions. It is important that the patient understands that, even at an unconscious level, there may be objections to the pregnancy, and that those objections may manifest in attempts to void the pregnancy.

Inquiry and resolution Having identified possible roots of the nausea, rational discussion, coupled with possible reframing and decision-making, should take place prior to trance work. Then, in trance, the decisions and opinions reached consciously are tested for unconscious acceptability and if accepted, integrated there. If problems are apparent, using brief techniques such as ideomotor responses is effective. Subliminal Therapy can also be employed effectively. If relief is not obtained by this procedure, it will be necessary to uncover unconscious influences that are causing the problem.

Testing nausea control While the patient is in trance, she should be guided to experience a bit of nausea through direct suggestion, and then guided away from the experience, teaching her cues for future use on her own. Progressively increasing the degree of nausea through subsequent suggestions, followed by removing the nausea, will convince her that such control is possible, knowing that whatever she can bring on, she can take away. The next step is to teach her to do it herself.

Suggestions in trance Each of the following suggestions should be made, using language and emphasis appropriate for the patient, but only after the above housekeeping tasks have been accomplished:

- *The nausea is no longer functional. It is neither needed, nor is it desired. It is okay for all nausea to cease, not only for the moment, but also for the future of this pregnancy.*

- *The issues that have caused the nausea have been identified, addressed, and resolved in the best way possible, and you have made the best decisions possible. It's okay, now, for the nausea to cease.*

- *It is now okay for a balance of functioning to be restored.*

- *Comments heard from others, however well intended, which might have caused concern, are to be unheeded; they are to be treated as if they had never been heard. After all, you know better than they what is best for you.*

Use of imagery The mother-to-be can be guided to engage her imagination, to privately imagine the course of her pregnancy just as she would want it to be – free of nausea and of irrelevant concerns, free to be joyful and optimistic. After all, there is nothing more profound than the creation of life.

Birthing

There is no question that stress impacts physiology. Therefore, how would it *not* be possible for the stress of an impending delivery to adversely impact that delivery?

Three phases are involved in a comprehensive preparation for delivery that will ease the delivery and minimize discomfort. First, it is necessary to ensure that the mother-to-be is informed about the process of delivery in an optimistic and positive way. Second, there should be a thorough "housekeeping" effort, in which both conscious and unconscious concerns are identified and then examined under the light of objective consideration as to reality and importance. Having accomplished the first and second objectives, the mother-to-be should be trained in the self-use of hypnosis for application at the time of delivery. The second and third phases are addressed here.

The training afforded under the "Bradley" method of delivery preparation is the best available for satisfaction of Step 1. Although the "Lamaze" training is the most commonly used, it is problematic in one respect: teaching the use of "panting" as a means of pain control. This is, in itself, a rather profound, covert suggestion to experience pain. In fact, in his book *Painless Childbirth (1965)*, Fernand Lamaze, M.D., described training that is far different from that which is taught in his name.

Housekeeping
These steps will serve to set the stage for the hypnotic work.

1. Discuss consciously identified concerns, whether they are seen as justified or not. Inform the patient regarding these concerns and reassure her to the extent possible, perhaps encouraging further inquiry about other issues with assistance from the attending physician. Discuss the "Lamaze" and "Bradley" birthing techniques, such that informed choices can be made. Offer new perspectives regarding the identified fears and test for validity by discussion. Inform the patient about the translation of fear into bodily tension, and the consequent effects. Define and reinforce those coping resources that are available to the patient.

2. Identify negative expectancies/beliefs about the delivery. Present them from a new perspective and test for validity as she perceives them, by discussion. Discuss the influence of beliefs, as well as emotions, on physiology. Consider possible influences derived from her personal birth experience.

3. Teach the patient self-hypnosis and instruct her in autosuggestion techniques.

4. Use Subliminal Therapy to comprehensively identify and resolve concerns that have not been recognized consciously. In order to assist Centrum, mention possible fears to be sensitive to: the fear of pain, of having a deformed child, the unknown, etc.

Preparation for delivery

If possible and prudent, accomplish the following steps in the presence of, and with the assistance of, the father of the baby.

1. Guide the patient to experience trance, then guide her through several compounding exercises to ensure adequate depth.

2. Attach hypnosis to sleep, as described in Chapter 11.
    Guide the patient to experience anesthesia or analgesia, as possible, perhaps by numbing a hand. Then, by squeezing or pinching her hand, test the numbness to her satisfaction. Offer detailed suggestions about the delivery process, including, at a minimum, the following essential points:

- The concept of a "comfortable" delivery, including examples.
- General comfort about the entire delivery process (conceptually compare it to a bowel movement).
- Belief in a positive outcome.
- Protection against the influence of uninformed comments by staff and others.
- Protection against surprise.
- Automatic/cued experience of anesthesia/analgesia.
- Awareness of, and interest in, the entire delivery process.
- Contractions to open the cervix, each helping to carry the baby forward, each to carry the mother rapidly toward release of the child, because the muscles "above" work hard and efficiently, whereas the muscles "below" are flaccid and yielding. In this way, the process is easy on mother and baby, and it all happens in such a short period of time. Each contraction is felt only in a pleasant way.
- The ability to control body and mind (i.e., the experience).
- The ability to participate and cooperate as necessary.
- The experience of pleasure, and even amazement, at her own success.
- Insulation from negative interpretation of remarks by others in attendance, including insulation from the element of surprise, so that the effect of such remarks will be to deepen the hypnotic experience.
- Indifference to the episiotomy and its repair.

3. Post-delivery suggestions, should include at least the following:
   - Feel wonderful.
   - Find yourself smiling.
   - Feel strong, even refreshed.
   - Feel hungry.
   - Recovery will be rapid and sure because of the lack of tension.
   - If you wish to nurse, the supply of nourishing milk will be plentiful when needed.
   - If you do not wish to nurse, your breasts will produce only a minimal amount of milk and will cease production altogether within a very few hours.

Ocular Correction

I am not aware of any published literature regarding our ability to influence the more essential functions of eye muscles by premeditated means. Yet, I am convinced it is possible to do so. The muscles of the eye are smooth muscles, controlled by a combination of sophisticated, unconscious thoughts and volition. We are able to directly and constructively influence other systems of smooth muscle, so why not these? The essential muscles of the eye shape the lenses to focus an image on the retina. Those same muscles can distort the lenses, creating astigmatism and other problems.

We are aware of the action of smooth muscle in coordinating, rotating and focusing the eyes. We are aware of the tunneling of vision in response to emotions such as fear. It could well be that lasting conditioning of the control systems regulating those muscles might be responsive to emotional experience as well. In my practice alone, I have had three patients discard their glasses in the course of therapy, even though that problem had not been directly addressed. Research is clearly needed here.

Oncology Applications

In battling cancer, the oncologist unleashes an arsenal of poisonous medications and locally exposes the patient to radiation levels far beyond those tolerable by the human body as a whole. All of this venom is focused on the cancer itself, but there is damage to healthy tissue as well. In the worst cases, side-effects range from nausea to nerve degeneration, and from loss of hair to loss of life.

Compounding the physiological effects of the treatment itself is the concomitant compromise in physical functioning due to psychological factors. Patients may react in fear, or depression, or by abandoning hope, all of which have negative impact on physiology. Thus, psychological treatment can alleviate suffering and enhance the probability of recovery.

By divorcing the patient's awareness from negative emotional influence, the trauma of treatment is eased, optimistic attitude development is promoted, and many believe the patient's prognosis is significantly improved. If only the patient's comfort is improved, it is worth doing: if other benefits accrue, so much the better. Moreover, there is no risk in engaging such treatment.

A growing population of clinicians believes psychological factors may be capable of *causing* cancer and other insidious diseases. The expanding field of psychoneuroimmunology is a reflection of a shift in the way of thinking about diseases in general. Many cases of spontaneous remission of cancer have been reported in the literature, and the phenomenon of such remission is not explainable within the medical model. The reduction in size or complete elimination of "growths" such as tumors and warts in the body in response to hypnotic suggestion, is also persuasive evidence of the authority of mental influence to alter physical condition.

We still have much to learn about diseases and their treatment, as we become more and more clear about the role of mental functioning at both the causal and treatment levels. Hypnosis will play a vital role in studying both ends of that spectrum as you, the health professional, expand your use of this phenomenon.

Pain Management

> *Pain is all about perception.*
> *Since hypnosis can control perception,*
> *Hypnosis can control pain.*

No application of hypnosis has received more interest and attention than pain relief. The capacity of the mind to not perceive a stimulus, regardless of the sense being stimulated, is at once dramatic and awe-inspiring. We have the capacity to selectively hear, see, taste, smell and feel. Or, we can selectively attune ourselves to be exquisitely sensitive to a stimulus. We demonstrate all of these capacities in various situations in life, sometimes without conscious awareness at the time, such awareness coming only in retrospect. The trance state of hypnosis, with its attendant capacities of selective attention, dissociation, and concentration, provides a medium to guide our perceptions in ways that can relieve pain that is of either physical or mental etiology. We don't really understand a great deal about the mechanism whereby such relief happens, yet it happens, and we can influence its course. As noted by Bowers

(1976) and Watkins (1978), the physiological responses to pain, as measured by heart rate and galvanic skin resistance readings, do not change with either chemical or hypnotic analgesia, yet the patient is subjectively relieved of pain. The phenomenon of relief of phantom limb pain by hypnotic suggestion is also informative. This section is about how to exercise mental capacities in working with patients in pain.

General Observations

As my first observation, I agree with Dr. Robert Magnuson (1984) that when using hypnosis, it's easier to deal with pain having physical origin, than with pain of psychological etiology. When considering treatment by "mental" means, the patient presenting a situation in which recent physical injury has been experienced can likely be treated by simple, direct, symptomatic suggestion, either overtly or covertly administered. On the other hand, the patient who has been in pain for a sufficient length of time to have accumulated associated secondary gain must resolve the secondary gain before effective relief can be achieved. Whether the gain is rational, such as a way of getting attention, or appears irrational, such as self-punishment for some act committed, it must be identified and resolved. Thus, intervention may be as simple as a covert suggestion, or as complex as an analysis of the psychological meaning, purpose, or function of the pain.

Older people are excellent subjects for hypnotic intervention, as are children. However, any traumatized person (adult or child) is in a state of trance, waiting and eager for suggestions for relief. If, additionally, the person is frightened, or in some other state of intense emotion, he or she is even more highly suggestible. It is the function of the clinician to offer guidance in the direction of comfort and rapid healing.

The clinician who uses a formal induction will find that pre-induction suggestions are just as important as those offered during trance. Those unplanned comments offered in the course of taking a history might have stronger impact than the planned suggestions. Moreover, suggestions are implicit in the situation, not just communicated by words. The suggestions offered through words, and implied by actions, carry into the trance state, and the expectation of outcome held by the therapist is covertly communicated. Fortunately, those expectations will probably become the expectation of the patient and, as I have stated, expectation determines outcome.

The concept of somatization is not abstract theory; it is real and viable. People experience all manner of discomfort as a consequence of mental activity, devoid of physical stimulus. Headaches, backaches, stomachaches, and even toothaches can be psychogenic. Moreover, depression, anxiety or psychosis can contribute to the intensity of pain, even though its basis is pathogenic. This being so, it follows that the preferable treatment for psychogenic pain is psychological. Yet, there is a problem here: how to differentiate between psychogenic and pathogenic pain. Fortunately, competent medical examination can rule out pathology and, regardless of etiology, relief from pain is in the best interest of the patient.

Words, regardless of how they are used, can bring up reactions and memories. These reactions and memories will, in turn, influence experience. It is therefore very important to use words that communicate desired, rather than undesired, experience. Words such as *sharp, pain, vomit* and *cut*, connote distress and should be avoided. Words such as *discomfort, incision,* and *hunger* (the antithesis of nausea) can be offered with equal ease and without the negative suggestion implicit in the other words. To say, "You may experience pain" is far different from saying, "You may experience some discomfort." To suggest rousing "with a feeling of hunger" is far better than to suggest rousing "without having to vomit." The mind seems to unconsciously lock onto dramatic words, whether they are negative or positive in intent. This is covert hypnosis.

As a result of hypnotic suggestions, pain may be totally relieved or may only be modified to the extent that it does not bother the patient. Therefore, therapists should not insist that relief be total and, if it happens that way, so much the better. In many cases, there will be strong resistance to "totally" relieving the pain. If the pain is psychogenic, it is serving some purpose, and unless and until that purpose is fully resolved, total relief will be denied. On the other hand, the clinician can often bargain with the unconscious, offering benefits in exchange for limiting pain. Again, the inventiveness of the clinician comes into play.

Often the experience of trance, in and of itself, without verbalized suggestion, allows the patient to experience the alleviation of discomfort.

Chemo-anesthesia is consistently more effective if the patient is relaxed in body and mind. The amount of such medication can be significantly reduced when there is appropriate preparation.

Post-surgical pain is largely due to muscle spasm. Hypnotic trance, with its characteristic muscular relaxation, can be remarkably effective in relaxing such spasms, as well as in relieving the cramps, kinks, pains, and itching associated with rigid casts. Both skeletal and smooth muscle systems of the body are permitted to relax, to function in isolation from emotional influence, in the trance state.

Too much emphasis is placed on the importance of hypnotic "depth." The degree of rapport between the clinician and the patient is far more important. We have no objective way to measure depth anyway.

Although hypnosis has been used as the sole anesthetic in a wide variety of surgical procedures, its use as an adjunct to such procedures is more common.

Virtually all painful experiences are accompanied by emotional reaction of some kind. To the extent such reaction is present, it will likely exacerbate the pain by causing muscle spasms, hypersensitivity to the stimulus, or by other means. Relief of such emotional reaction can therefore relieve pain.

Acute versus Chronic Pain

In considering various treatment approaches in this book, I have somewhat arbitrarily divided pain into two classifications: acute and chronic. A more pragmatically accurate classification might be based on differentiating between situations in which secondary gain is present versus when it is absent.

Treatment of Acute Pain

Several hypnotic phenomena can be employed in treating acute pain:

- Relaxation. To the extent a person in pain is able to relax his or her body, the pain will ease to some degree. Moreover, relaxation can be accomplished by many means, but is perhaps most effectively accomplished in trance. Muscular relaxation is an intrinsic accompaniment of all of the following techniques.

- Dissociation. At any given moment, we cannot consciously think about more than one "thing" at a time. If we attend to "this" sensation, we cannot simultaneously attend to "that" sensation. We can, of course, jump back and forth between the two, creating the impression of duality, but conscious awareness of only one thing can be present in any one instant. Therefore, if the person in pain can be distracted from immediate self-awareness, the sensation of pain is avoided.

This seemingly simplistic concept is also highly effective. Mothers have instinctively known and utilized the principle from the beginning of time. Additionally, clinicians who have a good bedside manner, in addition to those familiar with hypnotic techniques, employ the principle to the benefit of their patients. The power of imagination should not be underestimated, and how better to augment that power than through hypnosis? Our imagination is the most powerful influence we have on the way we experience life. Hypnosis enhances that ability and helps channel it toward positive experience.

You might suggest:

> *If a large, fierce and angry dog were to enter the room right now, and were to stare malevolently at you – obviously about to attack you – your attention would be so intensely focused on the dog that you would have no awareness of anything else. This is an example of the ability we have to perceive one thing and, in so doing, not perceive something else. By focusing your attention on the feelings you are experiencing in your hand – or that pleasant and safe place you*

> *create in your imagination – you will find you will be less aware of all else, and enjoy a sense of comfort and well-being.*

- Time distortion. When we reflect on an event from the past, we can experience that memory in a fraction of the time occupied by the original event. In trance, we have the ability to compress our experience (in time) in the same way, and that can make it possible to reduce pain and distress. A suggestion relating past experience in which time passed quickly, to the desired outcome in the present, may have a strong influence.

You might suggest:

> *Perhaps you can remember a time when you were on a trip, and the hours passed very quickly, and you wondered at how quickly they had passed. In the same way, your mind can now allow time to pass quickly, and you can then wonder about how quickly it has passed and how rapidly you have healed.*

- Substitution. On occasion, the unconscious may be persuaded to allow a sensation of "tickling," or of "itching," in place of pain. For example, when administering an injection, a suggestion that, *"You may be surprised how little you will be bothered, even though you may be aware of a little tickle or pressure as I work,"* can alleviate the distress of anticipation as well as the distress from the actual injection.

- Amnesia. Anticipation is often a stimulus for pain. Therefore, it may be of value for the patient not to remember a previous, similar, procedure. The suggestion, *"When it's over, when it's finished, it's like it had never existed, like nothing ever happened at all,"* can redirect the focus of attention, permitting greater comfort next time. Offering this suggestion when the patient is in trance will be more effective than if it is offered out of trance.

Application Techniques

Warm hands In utilizing this technique, the patient is guided to experience trance and then guided to place his or her open hand in contact with the area of the solar plexus, holding it still in that position. After the patient's hand is in position, the following suggestion should be given:

> *As you hold your hand there on your body, you can be aware of the warmth your hand produces in your body, there, under your hand. Notice, as you continue to hold your hand there, the warmth increases and spreads, penetrating into your body. And now, place your open hand on that area of your shoulder* (or wherever the pain is experienced). *Again, notice the warmth of your hand, and notice as that warmth penetrates into your shoulder, through tissue, and muscle, and even into bone. And, as the warmth penetrates, it displaces discomfort, relaxing muscle and interrupting any communication of discomfort to your mind. Hold your hand there and tell me, do you feel the warmth?* (Pause, and continue when acknowledged) *And, do you feel the sense of relief flowing in and the sense of discomfort flowing out?* (Pause, and continue if "yes") *Then, continue to hold your hand there until you are as comfortable as you wish to be. I will know when you are comfortable when you remove your hand, permitting it to again rest comfortably at your side.*

As a variation of this technique, consider the following suggestions:

> *I'm going to place my hand, gently, here on your back, and I'd like you to notice the warmth my hand produces. There, now, do you feel that warmth? Good. Notice how that warmth flows into your body, how it spreads and radiates deep into tissue, and muscle, and even into bone. And, as that warmth penetrates deep into your body, the muscles all through that area are permitted to relax, and a feeling of warm comfort spreads all around. Let me know when that has happened – let me know when you are experiencing that comfort…. Fine. And now, I'd like you to place your own hand there, in place of mine. I'd like you to know that healing warmth is available to you at any time you may wish it. Simply slip into this relaxed state, place your hand there, and notice as the warmth from your hand flows into your body, and with that sense of warmth, the sense of release and comfort increases.*

Glove anesthesia In this classic technique, the patient is guided by suggestion to experience trance and then guided to experience numbness in a selected hand, usually the dominant hand. When numbness is experienced, and tested physically to the patient's satisfaction by pinching or pricking, the suggestion is given that when the numbed hand is placed on the painful area of the body, the numbness will be communicated from the hand into the body, and the body will also begin to feel numb, there in that area, and relief and comfort will result.

The sensation of numbness in an extremity is easily generated in trance. As influenced by suggestion, smooth muscle restricts the flow of blood to the area and numbness is a natural consequence. On the other hand, it could also be the product of imagination. In either case, the effect is experienced and verified by the patient before testing on the painful region, thus providing significant reassurance of probable success, and an opportunity to reinforce numbness as necessary, before the last step is taken.

Clenched fist Calvert Stein, M.D. (1963) taught the use of a deliberately clenched fist as a vehicle for dissociating pain. In this technique, the patient is guided to experience trance and then guided to make a tight fist with one hand. The tightness is increased to the point that, by suggestion, pain in the afflicted area is transferred into the fist, and experienced in the fist, instead of in the afflicted area. Having accomplished this, the patient is encouraged to "throw the pain away" as the hand is unclenched and vigorously shaken in a throwing motion.

As a simple validation, the reader is encouraged to make a tight fist, being aware of the discomfort this produces. This sensation can become a distraction from awareness of other pain and thus the suggestion for transfer of pain is readily accommodated.

Specific dissociation With the patient in trance, offer the following suggestion:

> *One of the important things about experiencing trance, as you are now experiencing, is that your ability to concentrate is greatly improved. And, just as you can concentrate on something, so also you can concentrate away from something. In this way, you can be aware of any sensation – such as the sensation of pressure supporting your left leg – a sensation you do not usually pay any attention to. And, in this same way, you can choose not to be aware of a sensation – just as you were not aware of the sensation in your left leg before you paid attention to it. You can choose to be aware of your thoughts, and to be aware of what you are imagining,*

> *and in this way enjoy the experience of being in a place of safety, and of comfort, and of peace. You can go to this place, there in your imagination, and enjoy being there as long as you may wish, at any time you may wish to do so.*

Reframing This is an interesting technique that can be employed without benefit of trance in a formal sense, and the approach is impressive to both the patient and the therapist. Although I lack a satisfying explanation of its mechanism, I have employed it many times, even in social situations, and especially with children.

The patient is asked, *"What color do you associate with the pain?"* (Or, *"What color is the pain?"*) Whatever the response, the patient is then asked, *"And how big is it? Is it like a basketball, or a baseball, or a marble, or what else is about the same size?"* Accepting whatever answer is forthcoming, the next question is, *"And what shape is it? Is it round like a ball, or flat like a plate, or of some other shape?"* That is followed by, *"Is it solid, or is it hollow?"* and then, *"Is it warm or is it cool?"* then, *"What temperature is it?"* and, *"Is it light like a feather or heavy like a rock? Just how heavy is it?"*

When answers to these questions have been given, the attention of the patient is guided to be fully focused on the pain and the series of questions is repeated with the modifier *"Now."* For example, *"What color is the pain now? And now, how big is it?" And now, how heavy is it?"* The series of questions is posed, as the therapist patiently awaits answers to each question, silently comparing the second group of answers to the previous answers. Assuming the answers change, and they almost certainly will, the adjectives used will progressively define the pain in less severe ways until a response such as "It's not big enough to see," or "I can't find it anymore" is forthcoming. At this point the pain, too, cannot be found.

Row of switches and lights In trance, the patient is asked to visualize a room in which there is a long row of big switches, with lights above each switch. When the therapist is satisfied the patient is indeed clearly visualizing as directed, the suggestion is made that these switches are in the neural lines between the source of discomfort and the mind and that, by disconnecting these lines, sensations can be disconnected.

The patient is cautioned that he or she is to disconnect only as many lines as needed to achieve reasonable comfort, retaining enough lines for normal sensation. The patient is then instructed to go down the line, throwing the switches one-by-one, progressively down the line, noticing, as each switch is thrown, its corresponding light go out, and noticing increasing comfort with each switch thrown. By voice tone and pacing, the therapist encourages the patient to proceed slowly.

> *And, as each light goes out, you can notice a corresponding release of discomfort. As each switch is thrown, and as each light goes out, there can be an increase in comfort, an increasing sense of peacefulness and quietness, until you are satisfied with the level of comfort you are experiencing. Then, leaving the remaining switches on, you can rouse yourself and notice how good you feel.*

Magic circle Dave Elman (1964) taught that the patient can be guided in trance to create a magic spot on his or her body, within which spot injections can be received in comfort, *"noticing how little it bothers or disturbs."* The suggested spot can then be retained and used any time an injection is required. Kids, especially, appreciate having such a spot and are highly responsive to suggestions for it *"to be there."*

A point of distraction A person in pain may be so focused on the experience of pain itself that it is difficult to guide him or her into trance. In such situations, it may be helpful to provide an alternate focus of attention in the form of mild pain stimulus at a different location. For example, pressure of the sharp edge of a fingernail (or its equivalent) on the forehead of the patient, combined with appropriate suggestions, can redirect attention. The applied pressure should not be of such force as to cause injury; only an amount sufficient to distract attention is required. A few self-experiments should provide adequate guidance.

Treatment of Chronic Pain

Pain may have purpose that is not consciously recognized. In situations where pain is chronic, that possibility should always be considered, even if there is apparent physical basis for its continuation.

In such cases, the intensity of pain may be moderated by hypnotic intervention, even where complete elimination is not possible. It is probable that, in all cases, it will be necessary to address and resolve the underlying influence that contributes to the pain before relief can be accomplished by suggestive techniques.

The reader is referred to Chapter 5 for elaboration of the techniques available to identify and resolve the unconscious purpose or function of the pain. Like other experiences, pain has psychic dimensions that are addressable and resolvable. Should the pain have a purpose that is rationally considered to be functional by the patient, it can sometimes be restricted in some way – to certain degrees, to particular situations, or to specific times.

Should it not be consciously considered functional, and yet apparently considered functional unconsciously, even after attempts at resolution by analytical means have been completed, it may be possible to create mutual understanding between competing domains of the mind, thereby accomplishing the therapeutic purpose.

Treatment of patients in the final stages of life Despite remarkable advances in the pharmacology of pain control, there are always those patients who do not respond to medication, who cannot tolerate medication, cannot afford medication, do not have access to medication, or who for reasons such as religious beliefs refuse to take medication. These patients are candidates for relief via hypnosis and are generally excellent hypnotic subjects. They are motivated and, if in possession of their intellectual faculties, are apt subjects. It is not recommended that analytical procedures be engaged; trance plus direct suggestions for relief is indicated. The technique, "A point of distraction," described previously, may be of particular value here.

Treatment of patients in preparation for surgery or childbirth Anxiety or fear, with accompanying physiological reaction, is usually part of the experience of patients facing medical procedures. At least to some extent, such fear is justified and understandable; yet, in many instances it is exaggerated and unnecessary. And to the extent that it is present, it will contribute to general discomfort, inhibit recovery, and promote unhappiness.

Fear is the primary psychological variable that can contribute to the subjective experience of pain, even though resentment, outright anger, grief, and other emotions may also negatively impact the patient's experience. The first task of therapy becomes that of identifying all such variables, whether consciously or unconsciously present, and then resolving them by bringing them into rational, balanced perspective (see Chapter 5, *Using Hypnosis as an Analytical Tool*). This task, in addition to eliminating surprise via education about the impending procedure, can reduce or eliminate the requirement for chemo-anesthesia and can greatly improve the subjective experience of the patient.

Treatment of patients in litigation, or on disability, because of pain Don't treat them! At least, don't expect success if you do treat them, unless they are willing to forgo the benefits they may expect from the litigation or disability in exchange for the relief.

Some Possible Explanations for Psychological Suppression of Awareness of Pain

The use of hypnosis as an anesthetic in surgical procedures has been well documented. Its use in acute and chronic pain management, management of nausea in obstetrics and oncology, alleviation of distress in electromyography and other routine assessment procedures, and the masking of performance-limiting distress in sports has been widely substantiated. How to explain such phenomena? Short of chemical anesthesia, how are these things possible? Here are a few *possible* explanations. It's nice to have at least a theory to lean on.

Endorphins A class of peptides known as endorphins, generated in the brain, has characteristics very similar to morphine. All of the beneficial, pain-relieving aspects of morphine are present, yet there are no addictive, constipating, or other negative effects. Fortunately, it is economically possible to quantify the presence of endorphins in the blood, and so it has been possible to adequately demonstrate that suggestion can prompt the mind to generate them in unusual quantities. This mechanism may complement or explain other theories of pain relief.

The "Gate Theory" of Melzac and Wall In their book, *The Challenge of Pain* (1965), Melzac and Wall propose the theory that the mechanism of blockage of pain sensation is that of interruption of communication of neural stimulus at synapses between the source of pain and the brain. Whether this interruption is mediated by electrical or chemical means is not hypothesized in the theory. Nevertheless, by influencing unconscious thought process, as with hypnosis, such blockage can be caused to occur. The action of the endorphins is compatible with this theory.

Alter egos Helen Watkins and John Watkins (1979) have devised a technique of psychotherapy based on the concept of our having "other" ego states that can manifest in unexpected ways. They call their technique "Ego State Therapy." In their work with hypnosis, they observed that while an experimental subject reported no conscious experience of pain in a test situation, the suggestion of awareness by some part of the mind other than consciousness elicited a clear, vocalized response such as "You're killing me!" In applying Ego State Therapy, communication is established with each of the various states while the patient is in trance and are then "cathected" – that is, they are educated/reconditioned/reframed such that current needs are met by means other than by perceived pain.

Continuous specific amnesia Perhaps it is stretching the imagination, but another possible explanation for hypnotic pain control may be that we forget about experiencing it on an ongoing, continuous basis. We know amnesia for a hypnotic experience is frequently encountered. We also know that amnesia can be prompted under certain other conditions. Perhaps we forget the sensation of pain, even as we are aware of it, and so have no experience of the sensation.

Personality Disorders

Personality disorders may be genetic in origin, or they may be psychogenic. In the former case, management of symptoms may be improved by the use of direct hypnotic suggestions; in the latter case, the analytical use of hypnosis may be highly effective in the elimination of the disorder.

A patient presenting with the characteristics of a personality disorder may be in denial of the fact, or may be subjectively distressed by the condition. There will be no apparent clues as to whether or not the condition is psychogenic in etiology. The only route to differential diagnosis lies in the history of the patient, and he or she will probably not consciously have adequate information available from memory, suppression of traumatic memories being commonplace. Therefore, if the disorder is psychogenic, the use of hypnosis offers the potential for accurate diagnosis and the potential for treatment. A history obtained in the normal waking state will differ greatly from one obtained with the patient in trance, assuming responsible guidance is provided. Moreover, the history obtained in trance will prove to be more accurate.

Some clinicians caution against the use of regressive hypnosis in cases of Personality Disorders; I do not agree. I see these techniques as the only available effective treatment of the disorders. As I understand their concerns, regressive techniques might exacerbate the disorder by reinforcing the effect of original event. It is true that simply remembering any event will reinforce the effect of that event; yet, if the understanding of that memory is modified by intellectual re-consideration, the effect will change.

The key is for the clinician to consistently ensure that the patient is anchored in present reality and is reconsidering the recalled material in the light of present maturity. Abreaction should be strenuously avoided, with dissociated recall encouraged. While touching the patient in a convenient, non-threatening way, offer frequent anchoring suggestions such as, *"You are here with me, in this room. You can feel the touch of my hand so that you know you are here with me. You are remembering an event that occurred back then. You are learning about the effect that event has had on you in the past, so that you can change the effect for your future."*

PMS Alleviation

This malady, known formally as "Premenstrual Dysphoric Disorder," is a common example of psychogenic suffering. Women are all too often conditioned to expect the onset of unfortunate symptoms immediately prior to their menstrual cycle and solely in response to that conditioning do indeed experience the symptoms. The conditioning takes place early in life, usually accomplished without conscious awareness by the influence of a loving mother, sometimes incident to overhearing discussions between significant others. Since such conditioning takes place without conscious awareness, it appears to be a "natural" process.

Many will, of course, challenge my position that PMS is psychogenic. It's just too simple, and the symptoms experienced are too "physical" to be accounted for by explanations of mental influence. Yet, I have come to accept this explanation as the most valid because of the many women who have been successful in eliminating those symptoms by the use of hypnosis in my practice, often in just a session or two. The procedure detailed below will be effective in alleviating PMS in a surprisingly high percentage of cases.

As with many presenting disorders treated by the aid of hypnosis, in some cases the symptoms may be alleviated by simple direct symptomatic suggestion, as described in Chapter 1. However, in some instances it will be necessary to employ the trance state, or other hypnotic techniques such as Subliminal Therapy, to uncover and resolve causal influence. Both approaches will be addressed here.

Regardless of the approach employed, it will be necessary in advance to acquaint the patient with the concepts upon which the procedure is based. For example, the concept that the experience of PMS is psychogenic will be foreign to many, and these patients must be persuaded to be open to the *possibility* of it being true. Pointing out similar commonly experienced phenomena, such as the physical changes that take place during anger, or the disquieting physical and mental correlates of fear, may serve this purpose. The patient must necessarily be comfortably trusting of the therapist, as in all successful psychotherapy.

Procedure Employing Symptomatic Suggestions

Alleviation of PMS by means of direct suggestions that address the symptom directly is best accomplished through simple steps, introduced at some time *other than* when the patient is experiencing PMS. Completion of these steps may be all that is necessary to resolve the symptoms, even on a permanent basis; however, when time permits, resolution of causal influence is recommended as well. If completion of these steps is not effective, or if the symptoms recur in the future, resolution of causal influence by analysis will probably be required.

1. Elicit and record the specific symptoms experienced by the patient, both physical and mental. This information will be employed in Step 5.

2. Guide her to experience trance, and ratify her experience of trance by guiding her to experience hypnotic phenomena, such as hand levitation, or a pleasant, early memory. Then teach her how to re-experience the state at will (i.e., self-hypnosis).

3. Obtain permission from her to elicit the symptoms detailed in Step 1, with the understanding the symptoms will be short-lived and will serve the dual purposes of teaching the skill of removal, together with providing verification, in the form of personal experience, that such control is actually possible.

4. While in the trance state, and with her aid, select a cue that can be used at any time in the future, if it becomes necessary, to remove the PMS symptoms. Cues may take the form of the making of a fist, touching two fingers together, or the wiggling of a selected toe, to name just a few. Clarify and reinforce the purpose of the cue, which is to eliminate the PMS symptoms.

5. By appropriate suggestions for the onset of one of the physical symptoms identified in Step 1, guide the patient to notice the onset of the symptom and, when confirmation of the experience is reported, progressively guide her to the additional awareness of the other symptoms, frequently verifying that suggestions are being accepted, until she confirms that she is indeed in the throes of PMS.

6. Suggest that, when she exercises the previously selected cue, the symptoms will rapidly fade away and cease to exist. Then, encourage her to exercise that cue and request that she advise you when the symptoms have completely disappeared.

7. Repeat the process, guiding her to bring on the symptoms, and then allowing her to relieve them, as many times as necessary until she expresses satisfaction with her mastery of the skill.

8. If time permits, reaffirm, by ideomotor questioning, the suggestion that she is now in control of the symptoms and has demonstrated that control. Ensure the skill thus mastered is expected to remain in effect from this time forward.

Procedure Employing Memory Search for Causal Influence

Discussion of the resolution of symptoms by the identification and resolution of causal influence, which may include reeducation of the unconscious domain, is included in Chapter 8. The present application for the treatment of PMS is typical of many in which the undesired response was learned during an earlier experience, and can provide an opportunity for reevaluation of such lessons learned in the past, in the light of present, more mature knowledge. Understanding the event differently, coupled with reevaluation of the insight, results in a difference in the ongoing influence of the event.

After appropriate training in hypnosis, and after completion of Steps 1 and 2 above, the process to be used is explained and an agreement to proceed is obtained. Then, while the patient is in trance, guide her through the remaining steps, as defined in the preceding section, teaching her to relieve the symptoms symptomatically. Combining insight and personal experience of the symptoms under self-controlled conditions will likely result in elimination of the symptoms.

Procedure Employing Subliminal Therapy

In situations where trance seems unattainable, or when responses to suggestions for memory are not forthcoming, the use of Subliminal Therapy offers an alternative approach. The technique does not require formal induction of trance and, moreover, resolution of causal influence does not necessarily require conscious awareness of the process engaged in, or of the action taken, in the unconscious domain.

The following is a transcription of a session involving the treatment of a patient for PMS using Subliminal Therapy. All eight of the steps defined above under symptomatic suggestion had been successfully completed in this case and I decided to address possible causal factors.

Note:

Comprehension of the following transcript requires familiarity with the technique of Subliminal Therapy, which is presented in Chapter 12.

Having established the chalkboard as the means of communication, and having instructed the patient to respond by telling me only what is written on the chalkboard when I preface my questions with the name "Centrum," I proceed:

Dr.   Centrum, are you aware of your conscious concern about, and discomfort with, the bloated puffy feeling, the difficulty in breathing, tearfulness, and the other symptoms you experience just before your periods? YES

Centrum, are you willing to cooperate in an effort to eliminate those feelings and symptoms you consciously call PMS, and about which you are consciously concerned? YES

Centrum, are you in communication with those parts of your mind that have been causing the feelings to happen each month? YES

Centrum, do you agree those feelings and symptoms are no longer necessary and are no longer serving a useful purpose? YES

Centrum, please communicate with those parts that are causing the PMS. The first objective is the establishment of mutual understanding between you and the other parts, and then, using that understanding as a basis for further communication with them, educating them about present reality. Let them become aware of the negative consequences of their influence, and their lack of purpose in your life now, as an adult. Perhaps those feelings served some purpose in the past; however, they no longer serve that purpose, and it is time now to eliminate them. Persuade those parts to your way of thinking and let us know when you have completed that task by writing the word "complete" on the chalkboard. COMPLETE

Centrum, were you successful in persuading those parts? YES

Centrum, is any part of your mind now disposed, for any reason whatsoever, to cause those feelings to reoccur? NO PART

Centrum, do you believe you are now, and hereafter will be, free of PMS and its symptoms? YES

Mary, do you consciously believe you are now, and hereafter will be, free of PMS?

Mary   Yes.

Dr.   Mary, please use your imagination and project yourself into the future, into the few days just before your next period. I want you to use this as a test to see if there is any symptom or feeling of PMS. Of course, the real test is in the real world, but this can be a very good one for now. What do you experience, there in your imagination?"

Mary   No PMS, I feel fine.

Dr.   If you will now, Mary, at your own pace, and there is no hurry, please rouse yourself, remembering all that has happened and all of the memories you have had. Rouse up and open your eyes, feeling wonderful.

Mary   I was teaching and I was very, very happy!

Self-harming Behaviors

To the rational mind, self-harm seems unfathomable. A beautiful teenager, male or female, is brought to you by desperate and despairing parents who tell you that their son is cutting his body with a razor, or their daughter is scarring her skin with cigarette burns or stabbing herself with pencils or needles or.... Such scenarios can lead to confinement and hospitalization of the child and, unless treated by a clinician who is trained in the clinical use of hypnosis, treatment will likely be fruitless. Unfortunately, self-injury of this nature is not uncommon.

Psychosis is an immediate diagnostic consideration, but these patients do not often exhibit other symptoms of psychosis. They are fully oriented, able to respond intelligently, and are typically motivated to solve this problem that to them is mostly embarrassing (as opposed to distressing). When asked "why?" they will not have an answer that is satisfying, either to you or to themselves. They will probably be willing to talk to you about the behavior, their thoughts at the time and other aspects of the problem, but they will not understand why they are doing it.

In my experience, the most usual common factor in these cases is that the harming is serving the purpose of distraction, distraction from some thought or memory that is intolerable to them. Treatment is therefore directed toward uncovering that thought or memory in a way and in a setting that makes it possible to do so without reinforcing the negative consequences of the initial, sensitizing event. By taking advantage of the dissociation of emotion from experience made possible by hypnosis, the patient can be guided to explore the etiology of the behavior and to make more mature, constructive decisions about those events that have prompted the self-harming behavior. In using hypnosis in this analytical way, the patient is guided to experience insight, followed by rational reevaluation of that insight and, finally, to the integration of the conclusions reached. That basic protocol should be employed, regardless of the unconscious purpose of the behavior.

Sexual Dysfunction

No other area of the human experience is so fraught with psychogenic dysfunction. Moods, fantasies, expectations, and experience blend together to produce outcomes that range from euphoric to dismal. Neither males nor females can escape from psychological influence and neither is able to consciously control the orgasmic experience beyond setting the stage for it to occur.

Consider the consternation of the male who experiences erectile failure. Consider the female who desperately seeks and approaches orgasm without experiencing that release. Preorgasmia, impotence, vaginismus, erectile failure, frigidity, premature ejaculation and compromised libido, in addition to many other malfunctions, are all examples of problems that could possibly be caused by purely medical factors, but are more likely to be caused by unconscious, mental influence that is the consequence of prior experience. Moreover, there is rarely, if ever, conscious awareness of the prior, causative experience.

To the extent that such problems are psychogenic, treatment using hypnotic techniques is likely to be successful. These problems, like so many others, are the consequence of conditioning, and conditioning can be changed. Analysis, however, will probably be required.

Smoking Cessation

Having completed my doctoral dissertation in this area, I can speak with some confidence about effectiveness of hypnosis in effecting smoking cessation. I can say that if direct suggestive hypnosis (only) is used, there will be a short-term rate of cessation of about 70%. The specific protocol used doesn't seem to matter. However, within hours or days, that number declines to about 25%. There are many published reports indicating higher success rates, but I have come to believe that these reports are flawed because they report only the short-term success rates without longer-term follow-up.

If the analytical use of hypnosis is incorporated (preferably adjunctively to the direct suggestive use), the long-term rate of cessation is about 75%. Identifying, understanding, and then resolving the actual initial conditioning that was involved in forming the habit seems to be sufficient for long-term resolution in most cases.

With respect to increasing motivation to stop, my approach is to request that patients list both the benefits and costs of smoking, and to consider that balance objectively. Since emotions play such a significant role in such considerations, I will then teach them self-hypnosis, and guide them to objective consideration while in trance, thereby being protected from the bias of emotional experience. I feel at liberty to suggest additional items for their lists and, assuming that clarity follows, suggest that cessation of smoking is indicated. I will proceed first with the direct suggestive approach, and then with the use of Subliminal Therapy to identify and resolve unconscious influences.

It may be possible to use Subliminal Therapy to resolve barriers to *motivation*. In almost all cases, the smoking behavior is simply a conditioned response (accompanied by physical and psychological addiction). Subliminal Therapy is effective in resolving such responses. Only the psychological aspects of an addiction are significant; any physiological aspects of withdrawal are gone within a few days, and it's important for the patient to know that is so!

One last consideration: I require that these patients spend one-half hour with me in advance, no charge, in which I clarify the following:

- I set a fixed per-hour fee at my standard rate (no compromise here!).
- I make no promises.
- I *estimate* three to five hours will be required (the most I've seen required is four).
- I make it absolutely clear the work must be done by the patient, that hypnosis is not a magic solution.

Stuttering

Little has been written about the use of hypnosis in the treatment of stuttering, the most common of the speech disorders. Dave Elman

(1964) lectured on the subject very briefly in his course, and these lectures were transcribed and published. The earliest reference discovered is the work of Quackenbos (1908) in his book, "*Hypnotic Therapeutics in Theory and Practice.*" In it, like Rhodes (1952) and Wolberg (1948), he taught the use of direct symptomatic suggestion in trance as the treatment of choice. Cheek and LeCron (1968), as well as Kroger (1976), encouraged the use of age-regression; however neither developed the process adequately for marked success. *The Journal of the American Society of Clinical Hypnosis* is silent on the subject. My offering here is based largely on personal experience, which in some ways does not conform to more traditional theories of etiology and treatment.

I believe stuttering is a product of experience, not of heredity or genetics. It is a behavior that is "learned" at some time, in some situation. If that is true, then alleviation of the behavior must be a matter of "relearning," of reconditioning. How better to accomplish such reconditioning than by hypnosis? To buttress this view, consider the ease with which a subject can be caused to stutter in trance, a stunt often demonstrated by entertainers who use hypnosis in their shows.

The Etiology of Stuttering

If a child or an adult is placed in a position of intense emotion, and, additionally, having a desperate need to speak, yet is denied the ability to do so, stuttering may be a consequence. The situation must be highly emotionally charged, probably perceived as traumatic, and the individual must be helpless. Three cases from my practice come to mind in illustration:

- The patient, an adult female, was emotionally abused as a child by her overbearing father. She was watching her baby sister while her father was watching television in another room and the baby choked on a toy. She was old enough to appreciate the seriousness of the situation and went to her father in a state of panic for help. He was infuriated at the interruption and would not allow her to speak. She stuttered from the time of the episode until treatment with me many years later.

- A man in his mid-twenties had stuttered since the age of about twelve years old. He had been playing in the street with a younger brother when he witnessed a vehicle bearing down on his brother. He had just taken a large bite of food and was unable to expel the food in time to call out. His brother was killed and he stuttered severely from that point forward, until successful treatment with me.

- At about three or four years old, Tony was made to stop crying by his father in an overwhelming and critical way. His father apparently believed crying was not acceptable for boys, and was determined that his son would not do it. Other episodes followed in which Tony experienced his father in the same way but the first was the most traumatic. His father succeeded in teaching the lesson: Tony does not cry. Tony did, however, learn to stutter.

Although there are other illustrations of the etiology of stuttering, the basic themes displayed in these cases have been, in one form or another, consistently present in every case I have treated. In any event, a course of treatment using trance as a vehicle of age-regression to investigate causal influence is of service.

Treatment

As with the treatment of many other disorders, the treatment of stuttering involves the use of trance as a vehicle to uncover the memory of the causal experience, thereby affording opportunity to reevaluate the experience in the light of more mature knowledge and understanding. The patient is guided into trance, guided to remember earlier times when stuttering was apparent, and then is guided to remember the initial, sensitizing experience. Having that information available, the patient is asked about his or her current perspective on the memories and asked if continued influence is appropriate or valuable in current life. Assuming satisfactory completion of this phase, the patient is encouraged to test completeness of the work by "trying" to stutter now.

Suicidal Ideation

We have the capacity to commit suicide. We can do so by physical trauma or by mental influence alone. Some people believe we have an innate right to commit suicide, that no one else has the right to interfere. I tend to endorse that opinion, yet I am also acutely aware that we make decisions that are biased by our emotional state at the time of the decision, and that, if such a decision is reached, it should be reached responsibly, without emotional bias.

As clinicians, we are obligated ethically and sometimes legally mandated to prevent suicide in all possible instances. For me, the ethics of such a situation demand that I do my utmost to ensure the patient is able to function rationally and is, in fact, doing so. I have found patients to be able to comprehend their compromised capacity for decision, even in the throes of severe depression, and that they will defer suicidal action until the treatment has had a chance to work. In my experience, on all but one occasion, this approach was effective in preventing suicide.

If a patient is so focused on one issue that evaluation of other issues is not possible, it becomes the role of the clinician to interrupt that obsessive thought pattern in a way that will facilitate consideration of the other issues. For example, the mental process of a depressed patient is focused on the experience of feeling helpless and out of control, oblivious to values regarding others, to convictions about religious issues and to the possible effects of his or her behavior. In this instance, the clinician must prevent suicide by any necessary means, and is obligated to ensure awareness and consideration of other values held by the patient.

The induction of trance, overtly or covertly, is the first step. By virtue of the dissociation from emotional experience trance makes possible, the patient is better able to function rationally and to make objective decisions about life.

Surgical Preparation

The reader is referred to the section in this chapter on "Birthing." Except for the steps that specifically apply to birthing, the protocol is the same. Relieving anxiety, providing suggestions that guard against surprises, promoting comfort and absence of nausea, encouraging rapid healing, and ensuring the rapid passage of time all apply. The essential step is that of uncovering unconscious influences that might interfere in some way.

Tinnitus Relief

Tinnitus seems to be the consequence of smooth muscle acting upon the eardrum in such manner that hypersensitivity to stimulation is induced. The reported experience seems similar in nature to the process of turning up the volume of a public address system until feedback occurs; a resonating, continuous tone is heard that can produce marked distress and interfere with normal hearing. The key is to decrease the level of sensitivity (i.e., the gain), by relieving tension on the eardrum through relaxation of the smooth musculature that is stressing it.

Spontaneous relief is often obtained by simply guiding the patient to experience trance. The resultant release of tension in smooth and striated muscle may be adequate to reduce the sensitivity of the auditory mechanism, eliminating the cause of the feedback and, thereby, the ringing sound.

Offering pre-hypnotic suggestions in the form of explanations for the phenomena – along the lines explained above – together with education regarding the concepts of hypnotic muscular relaxation may well suffice. Training in modulating the intensity of the ringing may provide the necessary control. Provision of specific cues may be indicated, cues such as touching the ear or stretching neck muscles.

Wart Removal

In his classic work, *Hucleberry Finn* (1884), Samuel L. Clemens tells us how to remove warts. He had Huck find a dead cat, perform a ritual with it, and the warts magically disappear. Today, we do equally weird things and achieve the same result. If you think this is nonsense, you are misinformed. Wart removal is the most researched hypnotic application you will find in the literature, probably because the research is so conveniently objective in measurement: all you need to do is count the warts (Allington, 1952; Clawson & Swade, 1975; Cohen, 1978; Gravitz, 1981; Johnson & Barber, 1978; Morris, 1983; Sheehan, 1978; Sinclair-Gieben & Chalmers, 1959; Stankler, 1967; Durman et al., 1972; Tenzel & Taylor, 1969; Thomas, 1979; Ulman, 1959).

The actual mechanism of the wart's removal is best explained as the action of smooth muscle to constrict the blood vessels leading to the virally produced tissue, thus destroying it by anoxia.

One of the most astonishing reports of research (Thomas, 1979) involved suggestions to 12 subjects in trance, subjects who were plagued with warts over their entire bodies. The suggestion was that they would lose the warts on one side of their bodies, retaining them on the other side. Nine of the subjects responded by losing the warts as suggested, two did not respond at all, and one of the subjects got confused and lost the warts on the wrong side!

Another, more common approach is "buying" warts from children. The procedure involves the striking of a serious bargain between the child and the buyer: the child is given a coin in return for which he or she is to give the therapist the wart. The bewildered child will probably ask how he or she can let go of the wart, to which the therapist replies that there is no need to be concerned, it will take care of itself. The usual result is that the wart disappears within a few days.

Weight Management

The *Yellow Pages* in most cities list dozens of "hypnotists" who boast that they can magically get their customers to lose weight. There must be something to it because patients keep going to them, but my experience has led me to the conclusion that weight management is one of the most problematic of all presenting problems.

Direct suggestions, offered to a patient in trance, can ease the process of *losing* weight; there is no question of that. Yet, the time-honored pattern of resumption of weight after loss continues unless the psychological roots of the problem are defined and resolved. In this arena, hypnosis is of essential value.

Undesired weight may be the result of *eating behavior* that is prompted to satisfy some unconscious need, or it may be the result of an unconscious *need to be heavy*, in which case the eating behavior is simply a way to achieve the weight. In treating the first case, the needs must be identified, and there may be many. Consider that we learn to associate eating with occasions that matter: family gatherings, celebrations, religious milestones, and the like. Even in the beginning of life, we are held and loved and... here comes the milk! It is not surprising that we later find comfort and security in the behavior.

In treating a patient whose motivation to eat excessively is based on the need to be heavy, the focus is on identifying the nature of the need, and then finding alternate, preferred ways to satisfy that need, conceivably by recognizing the need as no longer being a valid component in present life. Perhaps the lesson of the past was that, when you are "big," they can't push you around. The message? "Being big is good."

Whether the basic issue is the eating behavior itself, or is the objective of being big, the conclusions reached in therapy must be integrated into the unconscious domain, as well as being acceptable by the patient consciously. In other words, the conclusions reached consciously must also be acceptable to the unconscious domain, and the acceptability is best determined by the use of the concepts of Subliminal Therapy (see Chapter 12). Questions of acceptability may be posed to Centrum with subsequent actions being determined by the response. It is often surprising to the patient to learn of those influences that were heretofore unknown, and yet make sense to them. My preferred approach to treatment is to begin by using Subliminal Therapy, resolving all identified influences favoring weight, and then employing suggestive techniques, including guided imagery, to achieve loss of weight, and then, to the degree possible, prevent the regaining of weight down the line.

My friend, Paul Kincade, points out the subtle, but potentially significant, difference between suggesting *loss* of weight, versus *getting rid of* weight. "What you *lose*, you can find again."

Chapter Fourteen

Applications with Common Treatment Protocols

The treatment protocols for the following problems are so similar that separate descriptions are unnecessary. In treating each of these problems, the clinician is advised to employ both suggestive and analytical hypnotic procedures, the sequence to be determined by clinical judgment. Although it is possible that direct suggestions alone would be effective, it is possible that protracted relief will require addressing the problem at a causal level. It is prudent to assume the problem is the consequence of conditioning, with its resolution contingent on identifying and resolving those earlier influences. Only the unique aspects of these problems will be discussed here, the specific treatment protocol being left to the imagination of the clinician.

Anger

In the uncovering process, look for mistreatment or trauma, without prediction of the age of onset unless revealed in the history. Ensure that the patient becomes able to embrace anger as a viable and valuable emotion, and that he or she understands that the task of the moment is to eliminate the exaggerated undesirable aspects of the anger, and not to eliminate anger altogether.

Compulsions

We could not function in life without automatic behaviors; imagine having to consciously control the act of standing up. On the other hand, not to be able to stop standing up repeatedly without purpose would be intolerable. Be sure the patient consciously understands the *specific* goal of the treatment, which is to eliminate the compulsive aspect of the behavior, not its natural functioning aspect. In treating this problem, you are again dealing with prior conditioning; treating it as such will lead to success.

Depressive Disorders

The pharmacological treatment of depression is based on the assumption that the symptoms are caused by a biochemical imbalance; therefore, treatment consists of using medications to restore that balance. But what if the imbalance is the *consequence* rather than the cause? We now know without question that glandular function is mediated by mental process. We know that our immune system can be compromised by stress, and we also know that we can, in trance, replicate any and all of the symptoms of depression in a non-depressed person, even to the extent that they subjectively experience them. These facts, coupled with my experience in relieving depression by identifying and resolving its psychological causes, have led me to the conclusion that the biochemical imbalance is, in fact, the consequence, not the cause.

Using hypnotic techniques, including Subliminal Therapy, to uncover and resolve the psychological roots of depression is the most effective treatment available. Yet in some instances, the depression may be so deep that masking it by medication may be required as a condition of psychotherapy. A patient suffering from an episode of major depression is not likely to be capable of logical reasoning, and so will not profit from an uncovering process. On the other hand, he or she may benefit from the experience of trance itself as a way to dissociate from the pain of depression. In the end, however, causes must be identified and resolved before actual elimination of the depression will occur.

Dermatological Disorders

The derma is sensitive to many influences, some imposed from without, and some imposed from within. To be sure, the manifestation is physical; for example, hives and other outbreaks are the consequence of glandular activity gone awry. But it is important to remember that those glands are mediated by smooth muscles,

muscles that are controlled by unconscious processes. Define the emotional root and the first step has been taken.

Eating Disorders

The focus of treatment in these cases must initially be on identifying and correcting the conditioning responsible for the distorted values held by the patient; resolution of the eating-behavior problem will not be possible without this step. As is the case with many psychogenic problems, the influence behind the behavior, which is held by the patient at an unconscious level, is not logically explainable consciously and therefore is not resolvable by rational arguments. Patients often recognize the irrationality of the situation, and yet stubbornly defend the condition they are in. Point out the inconsistency of one of the presented arguments, and if able to acknowledge the inconsistency, invite the patient to explore its roots, using hypnosis to do so.

Gastrointestinal Disorders

Our stomachs can take a terrible beating from our emotions. The system of smooth muscles that propels food products through the digestive tract is, of course, controlled by unconscious process. When these muscles are responding to an emotional condition, a malfunction can occur. Furthermore, if a physical reaction to some emotion begins, and that emotion is sustained over a prolonged period of time, a diagnosis of a physical illness may result. GI problems are among the most common of these reactions.

Insomnia

If no medical basis for insomnia has been found, and it has been a problem of many years duration, look for a situation in which a fear of sleeping was involved, or there was a significant payoff for staying awake. If it's an acute situation, perhaps the self-use of hypnosis with the suggestion that sleep will follow trance will be effective.

Phobias

Phobias are generally easily treated with hypnosis. This is so because their etiology is usually that of a single event rather than the consequence of an accumulation of influences stemming from many events. Direct suggestions are not apt to be effective, but identification and resolution of the initial sensitizing event probably will be.

Posttraumatic Stress Disorder (PTSD)

This is another name for symptoms that are the consequence of reactions learned in traumatic situations. The analytical use of hypnosis will probably be required, with Subliminal Therapy the procedure of choice.

Self-harming Behaviors

Self-harm equals self-punishment. The symptom is the abuse; the problem is that the reason for the abuse is not consciously known and the solution lies in uncovering the reason, followed by objective reevaluation by the patient. Hypnoanalysis is the treatment of choice and will almost certainly solve the problem.

Self-esteem Enhancement

Possessing high self-esteem is the natural state for humans. If absent or compromised, this is attributable to a life experience of a negative or perhaps traumatic nature. Identify the experience and resolve its effect – and self-esteem returns.

Trichotillomania

People shy away from those who behave oddly, and people who compulsively pull hair from their bodies are behaving oddly. Actually, it is simply a compulsion, the consequence of conditioning; in this case, it is the distorted thinking of childhood. There is a distinct sensation as a hair is pulled from the skin, and that sensation can be utilized as a distraction – as a means of thought-avoidance or as a means of self-punishment. Identify its function, guide the patient to reevaluate and reframe its genesis – and you will succeed in eliminating the behavior.

Part V

General Observations

Chapter Fifteen

Information Not Covered Elsewhere

*Because the structure of our bodies is defined by proteins,
and because the binding and releasing of regulatory proteins is
directly controlled by environmental signals,
how we perceive the world and threats to us actually shapes our biology.*

Judith Acosta and Judith Simon Prager (2002)
The Worst Is Over

Several important issues are presented here, issues that somehow did not fit into previous chapters, and yet may be frequently encountered by the clinician who practices hypnotic techniques.

The Covert Use of Hypnosis

Hypnotic phenomena are engaged in many ways without the subjects' awareness. Used car salespeople, physicians, and mothers all succeed in bypassing our critical judgment in one situation or another, and that bypass constitutes the essence of hypnosis.

In the clinical situation, where the patient truly wants to experience trance, and yet is apparently unable to do so, it may be appropriate to employ an induction that is not recognized by the patient. Since you are in communication, all that remains is for you to guide the patient to focus his or her attention on something – anything – and while attention is thus focused, suggest by implication, or in other non-obvious ways, a modification of the experience in some regard, even a minor regard. Then, assuming a desired response, progressively suggest other responses, gradually altering the theme in the clinically desired direction.

As an illustration, assume an adult male patient desires to experience trance, and yet is resistant to all known formal inductions.

He responds to your questions, indicating, for example, that his favorite pastime is golf, and so you ask if he has ever noticed how helpful it is to be aware of the details of the ball itself, when addressing it in preparation to swing. Chances are this would be a new thought for him, and so you have already moved him toward focusing his attention. Point out that by paying attention to the lettering on the ball, to its dimpled surface, and to its brand name, he will set aside tension that might otherwise be distracting, and that in releasing that tension, his mind, too, becomes distracted from any other awareness that might interfere with his objective. As you are talking, he will be following your suggestions mentally, and will thus be focused on complying. Then, point out that he will find this release of tension that happens on the golf course generalizing into his life, thus alleviating the problem that brought him to you.

My exceptionally talented friend, Steve Bierman (see Chapter 8), teaches that unexpected departure from conventional thinking patterns will produce an altered mental state. He will invite children or adults to focus their attention on that "orange circle square over there on the wall," and to keep their attention on that orange circle square while he completes the medical procedure required. In this way the procedure does not bother them. This is more than a distraction technique in that the mind of the patient is analytically occupied in an effort to resolve the irrational elements of the suggestion, i.e., the "circle square." Whether or not the resulting state of mind of the child should be defined as hypnotic trance is a matter of academic definition. In any case, additional suggestions for ceasing the effort, or relaxation, will result in a clearly defined trance.

The Effect of Surprise

An individual in trance is focused on a single pathway. It is possible to guide that individual onto another pathway, but the transition must be gentle to avoid arousal from the state.

Several events can prompt a subject to arouse from trance: a suggestion, voluntary action, etc. However, surprise can be the most effective if it is perceived as threatening. The following examples clarify this point.

- A man in the dentist chair, in trance to ease anxiety and discomfort, is sitting nearly upright when the dentist – without timely notice – abruptly lowers the back of the chair.

- A woman delivering her first child is using trance to expedite delivery and maintain comfort. In that emotionally intense moment when crowning occurs, the attending doctor exclaims, "Oh, my God!" actually referring to the beauty of the child, but misunderstood by the patient as meaning that something serious has gone wrong.

When this type of reaction occurs, the patient will immediately arouse from trance, losing its benefits in doing so. When interacting with someone in trance, the clinician is urged to maintain sensitivity to the effect of surprise, moving and acting cautiously and, if preparing a patient for some medical procedure, expansively offering suggestions to the effect that unexpected events will be easily ignored and will have no effect on the experience of the patient.

The Importance of Feedback

When a clinician offers a suggestion for a given response, it is important for the clinician to know whether or not that response is achieved. Otherwise the timing and/or direction of the next step is uncertain. If the response is a behavior it can be observed; however, if it is for a memory or other mental activity, the clinician cannot know without some other form of feedback. In this case, the only feedback available is by patient response. If no response is forthcoming, ask if it has occurred. To proceed, assuming compliance that did not occur, will result in loss of credibility, with both patient and therapist the losers.

On the Problems of Conducting Research in Hypnosis

The preceding sections highlight one of the major pitfalls in conducting research involving hypnosis. The application of hypnosis, whether in an experimental or clinical setting, is an art, not a science. Interpersonal dynamics, personal expectations of both the subject and the researcher, training of the researcher, history of the subject, and many situational factors are always active, and it is extraordinarily difficult to control for all these variables. Also, as Frankel (1988) expressed it (with respect to mental research): "The primary difficulty is that of establishing acceptable controls in research involving memories of personal significance to the individual."

If expectation on the part of the investigator is a significant variable in a study, as is often the case in non-double-blind studies, external as well as internal validity may be threatened. It is difficult for us to be unbiased in our approach; we typically want to persuade others to our way of thinking. Because of the highly varied, confounding variables in designing research in hypnosis, acceptable double-blind studies are unlikely to be conceived, whether addressing memory or any other phenomena associated with hypnosis.

Yapko (1992) identified nine elements that are significant to the accuracy of memory and are therefore significant to research design. In a well-designed study, each could be controlled for, and/or each could be assessed as a variable; however, simultaneous control of all would require a monumental undertaking. Yet, to not control for all threatens validity. The elements identified by Yapko are: competing stimuli, motivation to attend, sensory acuity, mood, expectation, intensity of the stimuli, novelty of the stimuli, meaningfulness of the material, and elapsed time.

Musculature and the Autonomic Nervous System

As described in anatomy texts, our bodies function by the action of three classes of muscles: skeletal, smooth, and cardiac. We have conscious volitional control of skeletal muscles; we do not have such control of either smooth or cardiac musculature; control of these muscles is vested in the unconscious domain – which may also control skeletal muscles, even in opposition to conscious desire.

Examples of smooth muscles include those muscles that propel food products through the digestive system and the "purse string" muscles that regulate the pattern of blood flow through the body by variably occluding the flow of blood through the arteries of the body. Other examples include the muscles that control the focusing of our eyes and the regulation of blood chemistry; our glands, themselves, consist largely of smooth muscles that mediate their function under the control of the unconscious domain.

The action of smooth musculature is largely mediated through the autonomic nervous system (ANS), and since it has been established that the ANS can be influenced by hypnotic suggestion, it holds that our physical state can be so influenced. Moreover, if hypnosis is a naturally occurring state into which we spontaneously slip on an ongoing basis, a state in which we are subject to inadvertent suggestions, does it not make sense that our physical health may be so determined?

Our bodies respond physically to our emotions. Changes in heart rate, blood chemistry, the pattern of blood flow in the body, respiration, and digestive process are among the possible responses. Is it any wonder that a prolonged state of stress can produce illness?

Is it any greater wonder that we have at our disposal the very instruments needed to reverse psychogenic illness? If hypnotic phenomena can be responsible for an illness, it must be possible to reverse that illness using hypnotic intervention.

The Authority of the Imagination

After almost 40 years of studying hypnosis and human mental functioning, I have concluded our imagination is the most powerful influence we have on the way we experience life. In some situations we may be able to control our imaginations and, to that extent, we can control our lives; however, in many situations our imaginations seem uncontrollable. We may obsess about something or become preoccupied with unwelcome thoughts or images or even musical phrases. We may imagine dire consequences that are out of proportion to the situation we are in, and thereby create unnecessary problems.

On the other hand, when our imaginations soar in positive directions, wonderful things can happen. Solutions to problems can appear and health can be maintained or restored. Athletic performance can be enhanced and academic performance improved.

The relevant message is that we can most effectively control the course of our imagination while in trance.

On Tape Recording Treatment Sessions

The general population may have too great an expectation regarding the effectiveness of using audio recordings to influence change. Numerous CDs are commercially available that purport to use hypnosis to cure a variety of ailments. Although it is true that we are suggestible in varying degrees and under different conditions, we are not uniformly suggestible, and the potential of using such material for creating change varies accordingly.

Those who are not familiar with the principles of clinical hypnosis often view the phenomenon in an impersonal mechanical way, as though all patients could be expected to respond to verbalized suggestions in the same way. This is, of course, a misguided assumption. The degree of integration of suggestions by a patient is subject to multiple variables, not the least of which is the patient's regard for the therapist as an authority figure. Therefore, we must not underestimate the effectiveness of established rapport and the personal presence of the therapist in offering suggestions.

Clinicians who wish to make use of audio recordings are advised to record at the time of the original work with the patient. As the patient listens to the recording later, many of the attributes from the original situation are recalled and the suggestions are thus more effective. Whether the patient listens to the recording in the waking or hypnotic state, while asleep, or while under general anesthesia, this "customized" approach works best. The clinician is advised to plan the content of the recording in advance, so that all essential elements are included as suggestions. The composition of a standardized script may be of value; however, it must be the clinician's own script, phrased and expressed in a comfortable, personal framework.

Distraction and Hypnosis

Distraction plus suggestion equals hypnosis. This is true because the distraction provides the focus of attention required and the suggestion provides the direction for response.

Hypnosis and the Law

It would be nice to say that the law is clear about the use of hypnosis. Such, however, is not the case. In the United States, the states and some cases the courts within the states, differ in opinion, legislation and in case law. By the regulations in some states, the clinical use of hypnosis is not considered to be within the standard of care; however, in these states the attitude is changing toward acceptability. The more significant issues in law are with respect to its use as an investigative tool in law enforcement and prosecution, hinging on the admissibility of testimony from persons who have experienced hypnosis as an aid to memory.

Even within the field of hypnosis, authorities have held differing opinions as to whether hypnotically refreshed memory should be admitted. A longstanding public debate between Martin Orne and John Watkins impacted legislative action in many states. A debate is still active between many responsible professionals.

Orne (1984) held that with rare and easily identified exceptions, hypnotically influenced testimony must be excluded *per se* (i.e., automatically). He also presented a Bayesian statistical analysis indicating that, at a minimum, more than 70% of diagnoses of hidden incestuous abuse are likely to be false positives. Finally, he pointed out several factors indicating a largely iatrogenic origin to the [then] current epidemic of diagnoses of Dissociative Identity Disorder.

In strong opposition to the opinion of Orne, Watkins (1989) held that *all* memory – not just memory obtained through hypnosis – is suspect, and to the same degree. Therefore, in forensic use, corroboration is an essential requirement and, moreover, our procedure of cross-examination is an adequate protection in all events.

As of the end of 2007, the law with respect to admissibility of hypnotically refreshed memory in *criminal* cases in the various states is as follows:

- Hypnotically Refreshed Testimony is **Inadmissible**, *per se*, in three states: Arkansas, Minnesota and Missouri.

- Hypnotically Refreshed Testimony is **Admissible with Safeguards** in 12 states: Colorado, Idaho, Louisiana, Mississippi, New Jersey, New Mexico, Ohio, Oregon, South Dakota, Tennessee, Texas and Wisconsin.

- **Pre-Hypnotic Recall is Admissible** in 20 states, with each defining specific provisions and procedures for protecting such testimony in the event hypnosis is employed for investigative purposes. They are: Alabama, Alaska, California, Connecticut, Delaware, Florida, Georgia, Hawaii, Illinois, Kansas, Maryland, Massachusetts, Michigan, Nebraska, New York, North Carolina, Oklahoma, Pennsylvania, Virginia and Washington.

- Admissibility of Hypnotically-Refreshed Testimony is **Determined by the Totality of Circumstances** in the District of Columbia and 10 states: Arizona, Kentucky, Maine, Montana, New Hampshire, Rhode Island, South Carolina, Utah, Vermont and West Virginia.

- Hypnotically Refreshed Testimony is **Admissible without Restraint** in the Federal Courts and in five states: Indiana, Iowa, Nevada, North Dakota and Wyoming.

The law with respect to civil cases is not represented in the above data, and it should be noted that, in effect, the restrictions apply only to the prosecution (i.e., only to witnesses); the defendant is free to use hypnosis without restraint, thereby establishing a double standard in the law.

Epilogue

In this book, I have presented the knowledge gained during almost 40 years of my professional life as a psychotherapist, a career of employing hypnosis as a means of helping people accomplish desired changes in their lives. In the course of those 40 years, I have treated a great many patients, patients have who presented with a wide variety of problems – far wider than I hear reported by my psychologist colleagues, who tend to specialize in given areas. This variation was only made possible by employing hypnosis, and I pass on to you the challenge of further developing this noble gift.

Herein, I have presented theoretical constructs that explain the phenomenon of hypnosis, pragmatic techniques of application and specific application notes. Hypnosis has been the focus of my professional life as a psychotherapist. I do not expect that many established clinicians, who have grown accustomed to more conventional modes of treatment, will jump their ships of therapy and join me in my enthusiasm. I can, however, hope to influence beginning clinicians to employ this uniquely effective means of helping people to change.

There is a growing acceptance of the clinical use of hypnosis by clinicians and the public alike, yet many accredited schools do not offer such training, which should be provided via core courses in every school of medicine and psychology. That not being in the immediate realm of reality, perhaps the impetus for further acceptance must come from the other direction – from our patients. When they are made aware of the benefits available, they will demand that kind of care, and clinicians will then respond, motivated by economics. This can happen only if those dedicated to the cause aggressively publicize its benefits; it will not happen if we do not.

In the medical world, hypnotic techniques employing direct suggestions are most commonly indicated because presenting problems are more often acute, and the hypnotic response needs to be only temporary. For example in medical practices, hypnosis is utilized to provide comfort during various uncomfortable procedures that are accomplished in a brief period of time. In contrast, in the world of psychotherapy, presenting problems are more commonly of a chronic nature. As examples, depression and anxiety often have a protracted history, with the current episode being one of a long series, and most presenting problems derive from past experiences. In these cases, at least temporary relief can be offered by direct suggestion; however, the analytic use of hypnosis greatly enhances the possibility of an actual cure. It is in this domain that I believe the greatest value of hypnosis lies. Let's cease wrestling with symptoms. Let's identify *causal* factors. When they are resolved, the symptoms will cease to exist.

Through the emerging fields of psychoneuroimmunology and related disciplines, we are becoming increasingly aware of the close relationship that exists between mental function and physiological response, including the genesis of many illnesses that were previously considered to be immune to mental influence. Hypnosis holds the potential of leading the way in the research, diagnosis, and treatment of illness, both physical and mental.

Hypnotic techniques, even if limited to the use of hypnotic language, will enhance the effectiveness of every clinician. Hypnotic language facilitates building rapport and establishing the required therapeutic relationship. It also augments communication, and the benefits accrue to the clinician in the form of patient satisfaction and referrals. Ultimately, perhaps of greatest significance to the clinician is the personal satisfaction experienced in providing more sensitive and efficacious care to patients.

Appendix A

Glossary

A Dictionary of the Language of Hypnosis

abreaction   Re-experiencing a prior event as though it is happening again, as opposed to just remembering it. The dominant feature is the inclusion of emotions.

allow   A gentle suggestion to permit without opposition, e.g., *"Allow your eyes to close."*

also   A way of connecting one suggestion with another in a binding way, e.g., *"As you allow your hand to rise, you can also allow a deeper trance."*

anchor   A way of relating a given event/sensation/time/experience with a desired outcome, e.g., *"Any time you might wish relief, you can touch your right thumb to your index finger."* A cue may be auditory, tactile, or both.

and   Smooths transitions from one suggestion to another without interrupting the flow of the message, e.g., *"You can experience trance at any time you wish and you can do so easily."*

as   Implies causative influence, e.g., *"As you lift your hand, your chest will feel better."* Also links one thing to another.

authority   A means whereby the critical judgment of a patient can be bypassed. The sole criterion is that which the patient perceives as authority. Authority is enhanced by trance.

become aware   A suggestion for awareness that implies conscious, cognitive awareness, as opposed to unconscious awareness, e.g., *"As that memory develops, you can become aware of the reasoning in your mind at the time."*

can   A permissive adverb to which unconscious functioning is highly sensitive. An indirect suggestion is, *"When it is appropriate for you to do so, you can become aware of the reason it happened."*

confusion   A state of mind in which suggestion may permit the focus of attention on a specific, suggested alternative issue. Useful as an indirect induction.

could   A permissive adverb to which unconscious functioning is highly sensitive, e.g., *"Although you could avoid the issue, you will find it easier to uncover the cause of the problem."*

critical factor   An expression coined by Elman (1964) referring to our ability to critically evaluate an issue. To "bypass the critical factor" is an example of its use as in an induction procedure.

cue   A stimulus that, when used in conjunction with a suggestion, indicates the time of execution of the suggestion, e.g., *"When you arouse, you will find it easy to relax."*

curious   Being curious is an effective way to avoid conscious thoughts that interfere with communications from the unconscious domain. The suggestion, *"Be curious to see what memory comes to your mind"* is a way to preclude conscious efforts to remember something, thereby opening the door for communication of the memory to consciousness.

deep trance   A commonly used description that is without precise definition. We lack the ability to objectively measure trance depth. Alternately defined as a level in which language is translated into internal experience.

description to prescription   One procedure for trance induction. The subject is guided to awareness of some set of objectively perceived sensations, such as awareness of the pressure supporting his or her hand or awareness of some sound in the background, and then his or her attention is focused on some non-objective suggested experience such as a feeling of lightness developing in the hand. A non-authoritative approach to induction.

discover A presumptive suggestion as in, *"You can now discover a feeling of numbness in your hand."*

even Affirms the antecedent, e.g., *"You can be even more at peace"* or *"You can be even less aware."*

feeling A word that is valuable in being ambiguous. It can be an emotion, a physical sensation or an opinion; the patient gets to decide, e.g., *"Take that feeling back in time."*

for a while Implies only a limited time; a suggestion to which the unconscious is highly sensitive, e.g., *"You will respond to this suggestion for a while, perhaps only for moments."*

for now Implies that the suggestion does not apply to the future.

forget to feel A suggestion for anesthesia, when used in that context, e.g., *"... and while there in that recovery room, you can forget to feel, and you can enjoy a sense of hunger."*

going Implies a transition from one thing to another, e.g., *"You are going back in time."*

hunger A covert suggestion for the absence of nausea, e.g., *"... and when you are next aware, you can be aware of a pleasant feeling of hunger."*

hypnosis A natural state of mind that we spontaneously experience many thousands of times in life without identifying the experience as hypnosis. Examples include highway hypnosis when time seems to pass rapidly, and, alternatively, the situation in which our attention is riveted during a crisis. According to Bierman, it can be understood as a refinement of everyday communication.

hypermnesia The capacity of subjects in trance to recall memories not available in the normal waking state.

induction Bypassing the critical factor (according to Elman). The translation of description to prescription (according to Bierman).

it   When used in referring to something physical, creates dissociation.

just   Means this and nothing else, e.g., *"Just watch"* implies "Don't feel."

may   A permissive, indirect suggestion, as opposed to a demanding or commanding one. Such suggestions tend to circumvent resistance, e.g., *"As you close your eyes, you may notice a certain feeling of comfort."*

might   Implies "might not" as typically understood unconsciously.

only   Means this and nothing else, e.g., *"There will be only an awareness of the sounds in the background."*

post-hypnotic suggestion   A suggestion offered with a cue for the effect to take place after arousal from trance, e.g., *"When the bell rings tomorrow, you will discover that you unexpectedly feel sleepy."*

pretend   An invitation to engage imaginary processes and the powerful influence they can have on the way we experience life.

pre-hypnotic suggestion   Those intended suggestions in addition to ideas, remarks and comments, that are expressed prior to experiencing trance, the influence of which is carried into trance. Such suggestions are often the most effective of all.

rapport   The intimate relationship between subject and guide which, at least in the clinical situation, is necessary to facilitate trance induction, and that facilitates communication between subject and guide. This condition of mutual respect and empathy is the clinician's responsibility to establish.

really   Implies casting doubt, e.g., *"I wonder if you really have the motivation to achieve your goal?'* Denies the antecedent, e.g., *"This time, really relax that arm."*

regression   Remembering the content of a memory without experiencing related emotions. Involves a form of dissociation from emotions and may permit uncovering of necessary information without the threat of re-experiencing the trauma.

rouse   A term used to indicate returning to the normal waking state from trance. A term that is more accurate than "wake up" in that the subject is not actually asleep.

sleep   A misguided suggestion for trance to be experienced. Because of the confusion it might generate, this term should be avoided unless actual, physical sleep is the goal.

that's right   Ratifies present experience, e.g., *"That's right, and now allow yourself to relax even more."*

trance   A hypnotic phenomenon. A mental state often equated with "hypnosis" that has characteristics of enhancing the authority of the guide and that makes other hypnotic phenomena possible.

try   Implies failure, and may imply the existence of an obstacle, e.g., *"… and as you* try *to open your eyes, you will find they are glued closed."*

waking hypnosis   An expression that refers to the responsiveness to suggestions that may occur without the subject being in trance.

when   A term that couples a cue with the content of a suggestion, e.g., *"When you are in that situation, you can rejoice at your success."* Also, links one thing to another.

while   A transitional term, e.g., *"While aware of your breathing, you can be aware of comfort flowing in."* Also, links awareness of one thing with awareness of another.

will   A term usually used as a gentle mandate that is stronger than a suggestion, but is short of a command. A direct suggestion. A word that can be a command if used with the proper voice intonation. e.g., *"As you slip deeper and deeper into trance, you* will *leave the discomfort further and further behind."*

Appendix B

A Brief Bibliography of Unusual Uses for Hypnosis

Accelerated Healing

Elman, D. (1970). *Explorations in hypnosis*. Los Angeles: Wilshire.

Moore, L.E. & Kaplan, J.Z. (1983). Hypnotically accelerated wound healing. *American Journal of Clinical Hypnosis*, 26 (1).

Anesthesia

Esdale, J. (1850). *Mesmerism in India*. Hartford, England: S. Andres & Son.

Monroe, H.S. (1912). *Handbook of suggestive therapeutics*. St. Louis: CV Mosby.

Birth Memory

Chamberlain, D.B. (1980). Reliability of birth memories: Evidence from mother and child pairs in hypnosis. *Presented at the 23rd Annual Scientific Meeting of the American Society of Clinical Hypnosis*.

Chamberlain, D.B. (1988). *Babies remember birth*. Los Angeles: Tarcher.

Cheek, D.B. (1974). Sequential head and shoulder movements appearing with age regression in hypnosis to birth. *American Journal of Clinical Hypnosis*, 16 (4).

Cheek, D.B. (1975). Maladjusted patterns apparently related to imprinting at birth. *American Journal of Clinical Hypnosis*, 18 (2).

Ipecac as a Soothing Agent

Wolf, S. (1950). Effects of Suggestion and Conditioning on the action of chemical agents in human subjects: The pharmacology of placebos. *Journal of Clinical Investigation*, 29.

Blister Production

Bernheim, H. (1957). *Suggestive therapeutics*. Westport, Conn.: Association Booksellers.

Johnson, R.F.Q. & Barber, T.X. (1976). Hypnotic suggestions for blister formation: Subjective and physiological effects. *American Journal of Clinical Hypnosis*. 18 (3).

Pattie, F.A. (1941). The production of blisters by hypnotic suggestion: A review. *Journal of Abnormal and Social Psychology*, 36, 62–72.

Breast Enlargement

Erickson, M.H. (1960). Breast development possibly influenced by hypnosis: Two instances and the psychotherapeutic results. *American Journal of Clinical Hypnosis*, 2 (3).

Nyquist, O. (1986). Breast enlargement by hypnosis: A self-concept variable. Doctoral Dissertation, Professional School of Psychological Studies, San Diego.

Staib, A.R. & Logan, D.R. (1977). Hypnotic stimulation of breast growth. *American Journal of Clinical Hypnosis*, 19 (4).

Willard, R.D. (1977). Breast enlargement through visual imagery and hypnosis. *American Journal of Clinical Hypnosis*. 19 (4).

Calming the GI Tract

Elman, D. (1970). Speaking on the soothing effects of rectally injected barium. *Explorations in hypnosis.* Los Angeles: Nash.

Contraception

Perry, B.J. (1980). Control of physiological phenomena via hypnosis with special reference to contraception. *Australian Journal of Clinical Hypnotherapy,* 1, 2.

Fasciculations

Overlade, D.C. (1976). The production of fasciculations by hypnosis. *American Journal of Clinical Hypnosis,* 19 (1).

Pupil Response

Erickson, M.H. (1965). Acquired control of pupillary responses. *American Journal of Clinical Hypnosis,* 7 (3).

Recall of Sounds Perceived Under Surgical Anesthesia

Brunn, J.T. (1963). The capacity to hear, understand and to remember experiences during chemo-anesthesia: A personal experience. *American Journal of Clinical Hypnosis,* 6 (1).

Cheek, D.B. (1959). Unconscious perception of meaningful sounds during surgical anesthesia as revealed under hypnosis. *American Journal of Clinical Hypnosis,* 1 (2).

Cheek, D.B. (1964). Further evidence of persistence of hearing under chemo-anesthesia. A detailed case report. *American Journal of Clinical Hypnosis.* 7 (1).

Cheek, D.B. (1966). The meaning of continued hearing sense under general chemo-anesthesia: A progress report and report of a case. *American Journal of Clinical Hypnosis*, 8 (9).

Erickson, M.H. (1963). Chemo-anesthesia in relation to hearing and memory. *American Journal of Clinical Hypnosis*, 6 (1).

Levinson, B.W. (1965). States of awareness under general anesthesia. *Medical Proceedings (Medise Bydraes)*, VII (11).

Selective Blood Flow

Bishay, E.G, Stephens, G., & Lee, C. (1984). Hypnotic control of upper gastrointestinal hemorrhage: A case report. *American Journal of Clinical Hypnosis*, 27 (1).

Clawson, T.A. & Swade, R.H. (1975). The hypnotic control of blood flow and pain: The cure of warts and the potential for the use of hypnosis in the treatment of cancer. *American Journal of Clinical Hypnosis*, 17 (3).

Conn, L. & Mott, T. (1984). Plethysmographic demonstration of rapid vasodilation by direct suggestion: A case of Raynaud's disease treated by hypnosis. *American Journal of Clinical Hypnosis*, 26, (3).

Tumor Remission

Gravitz, M.A. (1985). An 1846 report of tumor remission associated with hypnosis. *American Journal of Clinical Hypnosis*, 28 (1).

Wart Removal

Allington, H.V. (1952). Review of the psychotherapy of warts. *Archives of Dermatology and Syphilogy*, 66.

Clawson, T.A. & Swade, R.H. (1975). The hypnotic control of blood flow and pain: The cure of warts and the potential for the use of hypnosis in the treatment of cancer. *American Journal of Clinical Hypnosis,* 17 (3).

Cohen, S.B. (1978). Warts (Editorial). *American Journal of Clinical Hypnosis,* 20 (3).

Gravitz, M.A. (1981). The production of warts by suggestion as a cultural phenomenon. *American Journal of Clinical Hypnosis,* 23 (4).

Johnson, R.F.Q. & Barber, T.X. (1978). Hypnosis, suggestions and warts: An experimental investigation implicating the importance of "believed-in efficacy." *American Journal of Clinical Hypnosis,* 20, (3).

Morris, B.A.P. (1985). Hypnotic treatment of warts using the Simonton visualization technique: A case report. *American Journal of Clinical Hypnosis,* 27 (4).

Sheehan, D.V. (1978). Influence of psychosocial factors in wart remission. *American Journal of Clinical Hypnosis,* 20 (3).

Sinclair-Gieben, A.H.C. & Chalmers, D. (1959). Evaluation of treatment of warts by hypnosis. *The Lancet,* Oct, 3.

Stankler, L. (1967). A critical assessment of the cure of warts by suggestion. *Practitioner,* 198, 690-4.

Surman, O.S., Gottlieb, S.K., & Silverberg, E. (1973). Hypnosis in the treatment of warts. *Archives of General Psychiatry,* 28, 439–41.

Surman, O.S., Gottlieb, S.K., & Hackett, T.P. (1972). Hypnotic treatment of a child with warts. *American Journal of Clinical Hypnosis,* 15, 5.

Tasini, M.F. & Hackett, T.F. (1977). Hypnosis in the treatment of immunodeficient children. *American Journal of Clinical Hypnosis,* 19, 3.

Tenzel, J.F., & Taylor, R.H. (1969). An evaluation of hypnosis and suggestion as treatment for warts. *Psychosomatics,* 10, 252–7.

Thomas, L. (1979). *The Medusa and the snail.* New York: Bantam.

Ullman, M. (1959). On the psyche and warts: Suggestion and warts, a review and comments. *Journal of Psychosomatic Medicine.* 21, 473–88.

References and Further Reading

Allington, H.V., (1952). Review of the psychotherapy of warts. AMA *Archives of Dermatology and Syphilogy*, 66 (3), 316–26.

American Medical Association, Council on Scientific Affairs (1985). Scientific status of refreshing recollection by the use of hypnosis. *Journal of the American Medical Association*, 253 (13), 1918–23.

Assagioli, R. (1965). *Psychosynthesis*. New York: Penguin Books.

Augustynek, A. (1977). Recalling in a state of awareness and under hypnosis. *Przeglad Psychologiczny*, 20.

Augustynek, A., with Haynes, B. & Patrick, B.S. (1983). Hypnosis, memory and incidental memory. *Journal of the American Society of Clinical Hypnosis*, 25 (4), 253–62.

Augustynek, A., with Patrick, B.S. (1987). Hypnosis and memory: the effects of emotional arousal. *Journal of the American Society of Clinical Hypnosis*, 29, 177–84.

Bandler, R. & Grinder, J. (1975). *Patterns of the hypnotic techniques of Milton. H. Erickson, M.D.* Cupertino CA: Meta Publishing.

Bandler, R. & Grinder, J. (1979). *Frogs into Princes: Neuro linguistic programming*. Moab, UT: Real People Press.

Barsky, A., Saintfort, R., Rogers, M. & Borus, J. (2002). Nonspecific medication side effects and the nocebo phenomenon. *Journal of the American Medical Association*, 287 (5), 622–7.

Bellamy R. (1997). Compensation neurosis: financial reward for illness as nocebo. *Clinical Orthopedics*. 336, 94–106.

Beneditti, F., Pollo, A., Lopiano, L., Lanotte, M., Vighetti, S., & Rainero, I. (2003). Conscious expectation and unconscious conditioning in analgesic, motor and harmonal placebo/nocebo responses." *Journal of Neuroscience*, 23 (10), 4315 – 4323.

Bennett, H.L. (1988). Perception and memory for events during adequate general anesthesia for surgical operations. In H.M. Pettinati (Ed.), *Hypnosis and memory* (193–231). New York: Guilford.

Bowers, K.S. (1976). *Hypnosis for the seriously curious.* New York: Norton

Cannon, W. B. (1953). *Bodily changes in pain, hunger, fear, and rage; an account of recent researches into the function of emotional excitement.* Boston: Branford.

Chamberlain, D.B. (1986). Reliability of birth memory: observations from mother and child pairs in hypnosis. *Journal of the American Academy of Medical Hypnoanalysts,* 1 (2), 89–98.

Chamberlain, D.B. (1988). *Babies remember birth.* Los Angeles: Tarcher.

Cheek, D.B. & LeCron, L.M. (1968). *Clinical hypnotherapy.* New York: Grune & Stratton.

Cheek, D.B. (1975). Maladjustment patterns apparently related to imprinting at birth. *Journal of the American Society of Clinical Hypnosis.* 18 (2), 75–82.

Cheek, D.B. (1974). Sequential head and shoulder movements appearing with age regression in hypnosis to birth. *Journal of the American Society of Clinical Hypnosis* 16 (4), 261–6.

Cheek, D.B. (1994). *Hypnosis: The application of ideomotor techniques.* Boston: Allyn & Bacon.

Clemens, S.L., (1884). *Huckleberry Finn.* New York: C.L. Webster & Co.

Clawson, T.A., & Swade, R.H., (1975). The hypnotic control of blood flow and pain: the cure of warts and the potential for the use of hypnosis in the treatment of cancer. *Journal of the American Society of Clinical Hypnosis,* 17 (3), 160–9.

Cohen, S.B. (1978). Warts. *Journal of the American Society of Clinical Hypnosis.* 20 (3), 165–74.

Cooper, L.M. (1966). Spontaneous and suggested post-hypnotic source amnesia. *International Journal of Clinical and Experimental Hypnosis,* 14 (2), 180–93.

Crawford, H.L. & Allen, S.N. (1983). Enhanced visual memories during hypnosis as mediated by hypnotic responsiveness and cognitive strategies. *Journal of Experimental Psychology. General,* 112 (4), 662–85.

DePiano, F.A, & Salzberg, H.C. (1981). Hypnosis as an aid to recall of meaningful information presented under three types of arousal. *International Journal of Clinical and Experimental Hypnosis,* 29, 383–400.

Dhanens, T.P., & Lundy, R.M. (1975). Hypnosis and waking suggestions and recall. *International Journal of Clinical and Experimental Hypnosis, 23*, 68–79.

Dinges, D.F., Whitehouse, W.G., Orne, E.C., Powell, J.W., Orne, M.T., & Erdelyi M.H. (1992). Hypnotic memory enhancement (hypermnesia and reminiscence) using multitrial forced recall. *Journal of Experimental Psychology, 18* (5), 1139–47.

Dywan, L. & Bowers, K.S. (1983). The use of hypnosis to enhance recall. *Science, 222*, 184–5.

Echterling, L.G. & Emmerling, D.A. (1987). Impact of stage hypnosis. *Journal of the American Society of Clinical Hypnosis, 29* (3), 149–54.

Elman, D. (1964). *Explorations in hypnosis*. Los Angeles: Nash.

Erdelyi, M.H. (1988). Hypermnesia: The effect of hypnosis, fantasy, and concentration. In M. Pettinati (Ed.), *Hypnosis and memory* (64–90) New York: Guilford.

Esdale, J. (1850). *Hypnosis in medicine and surgery*. New York: Julian.

Erickson, M.H. (1937). Development of apparent unconsciousness during hypnotic reliving of a traumatic event. *Archives of Neurology & Psychiatry, 38*, 1282–8.

Erickson, M.H. (1960). Breast development possibly influenced by hypnosis: Two instances of and the therapeutic results. *Journal of the American Society of Clinical Hypnosis, 2* (3), 157–9.

Erickson, M.H., & Rossi, E.L. (1976). *Hypnotic realities*. New York: Irvington.

Erickson, M.H., & Rossi, E.L. (1979). *Hypnotherapy: An exploratory casebook*. New York: Irvington.

Erickson, M.H. (1989a). Basic psychological problems in hypnotic research. In E.L. Rossi (Ed.), *The collected papers of Milton H. Erickson on hypnosis, Vol. II.* (340–350). New York: Irvington.

Erickson, M.H. (1989b). Hypnotherapeutic Approaches to Rehabilitation. In E.L. Rossi (Ed.), *The collected papers of Milton H. Erickson, Vol. IV* (306–371). New York: Irvington.

Ewin, D. (1992). Hypnotherapy for warts. *Journal of the American Society of Clinical Hypnosis, 35* (1), 1–10.

Evans, F.J. (1988). Post-hypnotic amnesia: Dissociation of content and context. In H.M. Pettinati (Ed.), *Hypnosis and memory* (157–190). New York: Guilford.

Evans, F.J., & Thorn, W.A.F. (1966). Two types of post-hypnotic amnesia: Recall amnesia and source amnesia. *International Journal of Clinical and Experimental Hypnosis*, 14, 162–79.

Frankel F.H. (1988). The clinical use of hypnosis in aiding recall. In H.M Pettinati (Ed.), *Hypnosis and memory* (247–64). New York: Guilford.

Gheorg, V. (1967). Some peculiarities of post-hypnotic source amnesia of information. In L. Chertok (Ed.), *Psychophysiological mechanisms in hypnosis* (112–122). New York: Springer.

Gravitz, M.A., (1981). The production of warts by suggestion as a cultural phenomenon. *Journal of the American Society of Clinical Hypnosis*, 23 (4), 281–3.

Green, E., & Green, A. (1977). *Beyond biofeedback*. New York: Dell.

Grinder, J. & Bandler, R. (1981). *Trance-formations*. Moab, UT: Real People Press.

Hahn, R.A. (1997). The nocebo phenomenon: the concept, evidence and implications for public health. *Preventive Medicine,* 26 (5), 607–11.

Haley, J. (1973). *Uncommon therapy*. New York: Norton.

Haley, J. (1967). *Advanced techniques of hypnosis and therapy*. New York: Grune & Stratton.

Hilgard, E. (1978). *Divided consciousness*. New York: Wiley.

Hull, C.L. (1933). *Hypnosis and suggestibility*. New York: Appleton.

Jackson, E.N. (1947). *Understanding grief*. New York: Wiley.

James, W. (1890). *Principles of psychology*. New York: Holt.

Janet, P. (1907). *Major symptoms of hysteria*. New York: MacMillan.

Johnson, R.F.Q., & Barber, T.X. (1978). Hypnosis, suggestion and warts: An experimental investigation implicating the importance of 'believed-in efficacy'. *Journal of the American Society of Clinical Hypnosis*, 20 (3), 165–74.

Kline, M.V. (1955). *Hypnodynamic psychology*. New York: Julian Press.

Klienhauz, M., & Beran, B. (1984). Misuse of hypnosis: A factor in psychopathology. *Journal of the American Society of Clinical Hypnosis*, 26 (4), 283–90.

Klienhauz, M. & Eli, H. (1987). Potential deleterious effect of hypnosis in the clinical setting. *Journal of the American Society of Clinical Hypnosis*, 29 (3), 155–9.

Kroger, W.S. (1963). *Clinical and experimental hypnosis*. Philadelphia: Lippincott.

Kroger, W.S. (1976). *Hypnosis and behavior modification: Imagery conditioning*. New York, Lippincott.

Kroger, W.S., & Douce, R.G. (1979). Hypnosis in criminal investigation. *International Journal of Clinical and Experimental Hypnosis*, 27 (4), 358–74.

Kroger, W.S., & Douce, R.G. (1980). Forensic use of hypnosis. *Journal of the American Society of Clinical Hypnosis*, 23 (2), 73–118.

LaMaze, F. (1965). *Painless childbirth*. New York: Pocket Books.

LeCron, L.M. (1965). *Experimental hypnosis*. New York: Citadel.

LeCron, L.M. (1972). A study of age regression under hypnosis. In L.M. LeCron (Ed.), *Experimental hypnosis* (155–177). New York: Citadel.

Linder, R.M. (1952). Hypnoanalysis. In R. Rhodes (Ed.), *Therapy through hypnosis* (213–231). New York: Citidel.

MacHovec, F. (1988). Hypnosis complications: Six cases, risk factors and prevention. *Journal of the American Society of Clinical Hypnosis*, 31 (1), 40–9.

MacHovec, F., & Oster, M. (1999). In the best of families. *Journal of the American Society of Clinical Hypnosis*, 42 (1), 3–9.

MacHovec, M. A. (1997). Complications following hypnosis in a psychotic patient with sexual dysfunction treated by a lay hypnotist. *Journal of the American Society of Clinical Hypnosis*, 29 (3), 166–70.

Magnuson, R.L. (1984). Pain control. In Pratt, G., Wood, D., & Alman, B. (Eds.), *A clinical hypnosis primer* (173–186). La Jolla CA: Psychology and Counseling Associates Press.

Mears, A. (1961). An evaluation of the dangers of medical hypnosis. *Journal of the American Society of Clinical Hypnosis*, 4 (2), 90–7.

Melzac, R. & Wall, P. (1965). *The challenge of pain*. New York: Penguin Press.

Morris, B.A.P. (1985). Hypnotic treatment of warts using the Simonton visualization technique: A case report. *Journal of the American Society of Clinical Hypnosis*, 27 (4), 237–40.

Nyquist, O. (1986). *Breast enlargement by hypnosis: A self-concept variable*. Doctoral Dissertation, Professional School of Psychological Studies, San Diego.

Orne, M.T., Soskis, D.A., Dinges, D.G., & Orne, E.C. (1984). Hypnotically induced testimony and the criminal justice system. In G.L. Wells & E.F. Loftus (Eds.), *Advances in the psychology of eyewitness testimony* (pp. 171–213). New York: Cambridge University Press.

Pascal, G.R. (1949). The effect of relaxation on recall. *American Journal of Psychology*, 62, 33–47.

Penfield, W. (1975). *The mystery of the mind*. New Jersey: Princeton University Press.

Perry, C.W., Laurence, J.R., D'Eon, J., & Jallant, B. (1988). Hypnotic age regression techniques in the elicitation of memories: applied uses and abuses. In H.M. Pettinati (Ed.), *Hypnosis and memory* (128–48). New York: Guilford.

Pettinati, H.M. (1988). Hypnosis and memory: Integrative summary and future directions. In H.M. Pettinati (Ed.), *Hypnosis and memory* (277–89). New York: Guilford.

Pratt,G.J., Wood, D.P., & Alman, B.M. (1984). *A clinical hypnosis primer*. La Jolla: PCA Press.

Putman, W.H. (1979). Hypnosis and distortions in eyewitness memory. *International Journal of Clinical and Experimental Hypnosis*, 27 (4), 437–48.

Quackenbos, J. (1908). *Hypnotic therapeutics in theory and practice*. New York: Harper.

Raikov, V.L. (1980). Age regression to infancy by adult subjects in deep hypnosis. *Journal of the American Society of Clinical Hypnosis*, 22 (3), 156–63.

Raikov, V.L. (1982). Hypnotic age regression to the neonatal period: Comparison with role playing. *International Journal of clinical and Experimental Hypnosis*, 30, (2), 106–116.

Reiser, M. (1976). Hypnosis as a tool in criminal investigation. In *"The police chief" handbook of investigating hypnosis.* (1980). Los Angeles: Law Enforcement Hypnosis Institute.

Reiser, M., & Nielson, M. (1980). Investigative hypnosis: A developing specialty. *Journal of the American Society of Clinical Hypnosis,* 23 (2), 75–85.

Reiser, M. (1980). *Handbook of investigative hypnosis.* Los Angeles: LEHI Publishing Company.

Reiser, M. (1982). *Police psychology. Collected Papers.* Los Angeles: LEHI Publishing Company.

Relinger, H. (1984). Hypnotic hypermnesia: A critical review. *Journal of the American Society of Clinical Hypnosis,* 26 (3), 212–25.

Rhodes, R.N. (1952). *Therapy through hypnosis.* New York: Citadel.

Rosenthal, B. G. (1944). Hypnotic recall of material learned under anxiety and non-anxiety producing conditions. *Journal of Experimental Psychology,* 34, 369–89.

Schafer, D.W., & Rubio, R. (1978). Hypnosis to aid the recall of witnesses. *International Journal of Clinical and Experimental Hypnosis,* 26 (2), 81–91.

Sears, A.B. (1978). A comparison of hypnotic and waking recall. *International Journal of Clinical and Experimental Hypnosis,* 2 (4), 296–304.

Sheehan, D.V. (1978). Influence of psychosocial factors in wart remission. *Journal of the American Society of Clinical Hypnosis,* 20 (3), 160–4.

Shields, I.W., & Knox, J. (1986). Level of processing as a determinant in hypnotic hypermnesia. *Journal of Abnormal Psychology,* 95 (4), 358–64.

Sinclair-Gieben, A.H.C., & Chalmers, D. (1959). Evaluation of treatment of warts by hypnosis. *The Lancet,* October 3, 2: 480–2.

Spanos, N.P., Gwynn, M., Comer, S.L., Baltruweit, W.J., & deGroh, M. (1989). Are hypnotically induced pseudomemories resistant to cross-examination? *Law and Behavior,* 13 (3), 271–89.

Spiegel, H. (1997). Nocebo: the power of suggestibility. *Preventive Medicine,* 26 (5), 616–21.

Spinhoven, P. & Wijk J. (1992). Hypnotic age regression in an experimental and clinical context. *Journal of the American Society of Clinical Hypnosis,* 35 (1), 40–6.

Stager, G.L., & Lundy, R.M. (1985). Hypnosis and the learning and recall of visually presented material. *International Journal of Clinical and Experimental Hypnosis*, 33, 27–39.

Staib, A.R., & Logan, D.R. (1997). Hypnotic stimulation of breast growth. *Journal of the American Society of Clinical Hypnosis*, 19 (4), 201–8.

Stalnaker, J.M., & Riddle, E.E. (1932). The effect of hypnosis on long-delayed recall. *Journal of General Psychology*, 6, 429–40.

Stankler, L. (1967). A critical assessment of the cure of warts by suggestion. *Practitioner*, 198, 690–4.

Stein, C. (1963). The clenched fist technique as a hypnotic procedure in clinical psychotherapy. *Journal of the American Society of Clinical Hypnosis*, 5 (2), 113–9.

Stratton, L. G. (1977). The use of hypnosis in law enforcement: A pilot program. *Journal of Police Science and Administration*, 5 (4), 399–406.

Strickler, C.B. (1929). A quantitative study of post-hypnotic amnesia. *Journal of Abnormal Social Psychology*, 24, 108–19.

Surman, O.S., Gottlieb, S.K., & Hackett, T.P. (1972). Hypnotic treatment of a child with warts. *Archives of General Psychiatry*, 28, 439–41.

Tasini, M.F., & Hackett, T.F. (1977). Hypnosis in the treatment of warts in immunodeficient children. *Journal of the American Society of Clinical Hypnosis*, 19 (3), 152–4.

Tenzel, J.F., & Taylor, R.H., (1969). An evaluation of hypnosis and suggestion as treatment for warts. *Psychosomatics*, 10, 252–7.

Thomas, L. (1979). *The Medusa and the snail*. New York: Penguin Books.

Tierney, S. Unpublished poem. Printed with permission.

True, R.M. (1949). Experimental control in hypnotic age regression states. *Science*, 2 (110), 583–4.

Ulman, M. (1959). On the psyche and warts: Suggestion and warts, a review and comments. *Psychosomatic Medicine*, 21, 473–88.

Wain, H.J. (1980). *Clinical hypnosis in medicine*. Chicago: Year Book Medical Publishers.

Watkins, J.G. (1949). *Hypnotherapy of war neuroses*. New York: Ronald Press.

Watkins, J.G. (1978). *The therapeutic self*. New York: Human Sciences.

Watkins, J.G., & Watkins, H.H. (1979). Ego states and hidden observers. *Journal of Altered States of Consciousness*, 5 (3), 18.

Watkins, J.G. (1989). Hypnotic hypermnesia and forensic hypnosis: A cross examination. *Journal of the American Society of Clinical Hypnosis*, 32 (2) 71–83.

Wester, W.C. (1987). *Clinical Hypnosis: A Case Management Approach.* Cincinnati: Behavioral Sciences Center.

Weitzenhoffer, A.M. (1957). *General techniques of hypnotism.* New York: Grune & Stratton.

White, R. W., Fox, G.F., & Harris, W.W. (1940). Hypnotic hypermnesia for recently learned material. *Journal of Abnormal Social Psychology*, 35, 88–103.

Willard, R.D. (1977). Breast enlargement through visual imagery and hypnosis. *Journal of the American Society of Clinical Hypnosis*, 19 (4), 195–200.

Wolberg, L.R. (1945). *Hypnoanalysis.* New York: Grune & Stratton.

Wolberg, L.R. (1948). *Medical hypnosis.* New York: Grune & Stratton.

Wolf, S. (1950). Effects of suggestion and conditioning on the action of chemical agents in human subjects: The pharmacology of placebos. *Journal of Clinical Investigation*, 29 (1), 100–9.

Yager, E.K. (1985). *Subliminal therapy: Utilizing the Unconscious Mind. A book for my patients.* Self-Published, San Diego.

Yager, E.K. (1987). Subliminal therapy: Utilizing the unconscious mind. *Journal of the American Academy of Medical Hypnoanalysts*, 11 (4), 156–60.

Yager, E.K. (2002). Hypnosis in criminal investigation. *The Law Enforcement Quarterly*, published by the Office of the District Attorney, County of San Diego.

Yager, G. Unpublished remark. Printed with permission.

Yapko, M.D. (1992). *Hypnosis and the treatment of depression.* New York: Taylor & Francis.

Yapko, M.D. (1996). *Breaking the patterns of depression.* New York: Doubleday.

Yapko, M.D. (2003). *Trancework: An introduction to the practice of hypnosis (3rd edition).* New York: Brunner-Routledge.

Zelig, M., & Biedleman, W. (1981). The investigative use of hypnosis: A word of caution. *International Journal of Clinical and Experimental Hypnosis*, 29, 401–12.

Index of Names

Index

About the Author

Edwin K. Yager, Ph.D., is a Clinical Professor in the Department of Psychiatry, UCSD School of Medicine and a Staff Psychologist for the UCSD Medical Group. Dr. Yager also maintains a private practice in San Diego, California

Dr. Yager has studied, practiced and taught the clinical use of hypnosis for 40 years. Additionally, he is certified as a Consultant in Hypnosis by the American Society of Clinical Hypnosis. He is a Past-President, Fellow and current Board Member of the San Diego Society of Clinical Hypnosis and offers training under the auspices of the San Diego Psychological Association.

In the course of his private practice, Dr. Yager has treated several thousand patients who presented with a wide variety of psychological problems, as well as psychogenic physical problems.